# THE HYPNOBIRTHING BOOK

## Childbirth with Confidence and Calm

KATHARINE GRAVES

Katharine Publishing

First published in Great Britain in 2012 by:
Katharine Publishing, 50 Fosbury, Marlborough, Wiltshire, SN8 3NJ

This revised edition published in 2021

Copyright © 2012, 2014, 2017, 2021 Katharine Graves
The right of Katharine Graves to be identified as the author of this work has been
asserted by her in accordance with the Copyright, Designs and Patents Act 1988.

The author has made every reasonable effort to contact all copyright holders.
Any errors that may have occurred are inadvertent and anyone who for any reason
has not been contacted is invited to write to the publisher so that a full
acknowledgement may be made in subsequent editions of this work.

British Library Cataloguing in Publication Data
A catalogue record for this book is available from the British Library

ISBN: 978-1-911558-04-0

Hypnotherapy consultant: Archie McIntyre
Editor: Alison Candlin
Art editor and page make-up: Louise Turpin, www.louiseturpindesign.co.uk
Book and cover illustrations: Louise Turpin, www.louiseturpindesign.co.uk
Cover design: Alex Drewett, www.adrewittdesign.com
Index: MHB Indexing Services

Printed in the Czech Republic by Printo, www.printo.cz

This book is designed to provide helpful information on pregnancy and birth.
The information is as up-to-date and accurate as possible according to the author's best
ability at the time of writing, but knowledge and research evolve all the time. It does not
constitute medical advice or an alternative to appropriate medical care, nor is it in any
way a guarantee or promise of expected, imagined or actual outcome of labour or birth.
It is not a substitute for the advice or the presence during birth or any part of
pregnancy or labour of a qualified medical practitioner, midwife or obstetrician.
Neither the author nor the publisher accepts responsibility for any liability
or damage caused by or as a result of practising the techniques in this book.

All are welcome at KGH and our purpose is to support everyone during their
pregnancy and birth so that they have the best possible birth experience.
We are constantly working towards the language used being inclusive to all. KGH
supports equality and diversity and is completely against all forms of discrimination.
We support freedom of expression of a range of opinions. The KGH Equality,
Diversity and Inclusivity Statement can be found at kghypnobirthing.com

*My intention is that this book is the very best guide to put you in control and help you achieve the birth you want. It isn't perfect, and it never will be, but I personally, and everyone at KGHypnobirthing, want to be judged by the good that we do. Our goal is to cause a revolution in the care of birthing women so that all women can say that giving birth was the most wonderful and empowering experience of their lives.*

### ULTIMATE BIRTH RELAXATION

The free relaxation audio that accompanies this book is an intrinsic part of the KGH course. The tracks help you to prepare for the birth of your baby with calmness and confidence, under Katharine's guidance.

Download your copy at kghb.org/relaxation using the download code KGHAUDIO.

To connect with other, likeminded expectant parents, join our Facebook community by visiting kghb.org/fb or search for Hypnobirthing Group on Facebook.

Or follow us on social media

f hypnobirthing group
🐦 @hypnobirthing
📷 @kghypnobirthing

*To Archie McIntyre,*
*the unsung hero of hypnobirthing*

# What people say about KGHypnobirthing

"Beyond grateful to … Katharine for the inspiration, wisdom and guidance she shared, which empowered us more than I can explain"

*Ella Mills, Deliciously Ella*

"Katharine Graves is the Godmother of Awakened Midwifery. She teaches a very important aspect of feminism; how to honour and unleash (perhaps) the greatest power of humanity, the ability to create life and consciously bring it forth into the world."

*Russell Brand*

"My work with Katharine kept me calm and focused as my labour took a number of unexpected twists and turns. I felt well prepared and although I ended up having a C-section rather than a planned natural birth I found her programme helped enormously to guide me through each step. Baby Rae and I now happily listen to Katharine's meditations together – I think she recognises her voice!"

*Sarah-Jane Mee*

"This book provides expectant parents and healthcare professionals with a logical and holistic approach to pregnancy and birth, emphasising the importance of individualised, parent-led decision making. Knowledge is powerful, and the knowledge learnt from this book as an expectant parent will provide you with the confidence to approach your birth calmly, in control and able to advocate for your preferences."

*Dr Ellie Rayner MRCOG, Obstetrician, The Maternity Collective*

"KGHypnobirthing is well researched and supported by the latest evidence. This is what sets this course apart from others and why I chose to study KGHypnobirthing."

*Midwife and KGH teacher*

"The thing about KGHypnobirthing is that it works."

*KGH father*

"Helps your body and mind to sync and do what it's supposed to do."

*KGH mother*

"I recommend hypnobirthing to anyone who listens, it's a truly wonderful experience!"

*KGH Father*

"We honestly can't thank you enough and have recommended you to several friends. We are evangelical about the powers of hypnobirthing and definitely intend to follow it again when we have another baby."

*KGH Mother & Partner*

"Ever since he was born, countless people have commented on how calm and alert he is. He rarely cries and is incredibly watchful and 'switched on'. Again, we are sure that this is testament to hypnobirthing and the calm environment he experienced both in the womb and during his birth."

*KGH Mother*

"Katharine's approach to teaching parents is wholesome, nurturing, reassuring and informative. I left feeling so comforted, calm and confident."

*KGH Mother*

"From going from an absolute fear of birth to having no fear at all is the greatest gift I've ever received. Everything I learnt was put into practice and it paid off."

*KGH Mother*

# Contents

## RELAXATIONS AND IMAGES

To help you to find the relaxations that you are likely to use again and again in your practice, all the Relaxations and Images in the book are listed separately here.

# Author's note

This NEW EDITION of *The Hypnobirthing Book* has an extra 30% of material so there is so much more support and information for you than in the previous editions.

Birth remains the same throughout history, but the policies and procedures of maternity services change and even increase remarkably frequently. The principles of KGHypnobirthing are based on evidence and logic, and have been the same throughout history, but the course is changing all the time to respond to the procedures of the current maternity services and the latest evidence.

Even the World Health Organisation has issued a statement saying that birth in the developed world has become over-medicalised and it is time for the pendulum to swing back towards normality. Recently Prof Hannah Dahlen highlighted the fact that the rate of induction of labour is now 45% and ten years ago it was 25%, an increase of 20% with no increase in safety. Birth trauma is on the increase and what should be a joyful time for mother and baby has in many cases become a time of stress and worry.

Change comes from educated women who understand the implications of proposed interventions, the alternatives available (which may not be offered to them by the 'system'), and the potential outcomes. Only then can you discuss your pregnancy as equals with your caregivers and make an informed choice.

This is where KGHypnobirthing comes in. The course we offer is a full antenatal training based on evidence and logic. Thousands of women have now given birth using these principles and report the day their baby was born as the most positive and empowering day of their lives. But the epidemic of interventions and particularly of induction of labour, has grown since *The Hypnobirthing Book* was first written. This new book is up-to-date: for example, one of the new chapters is on birth trauma, with new relaxations to help release these negative memories from your life.

You are probably approaching KGHypnobirthing to achieve a more comfortable birth, and it most certainly delivers. But the effect on your baby is even more significant. People often remark on the serenity and poise of KGHypnobirthing babies, and it seems that these qualities may remain with them as they grow. Since they have not had a trauma to recover from they often put on weight straight after birth and sleep through the night sooner.

Birth is the most important event of our lives so the significance of KGHypnobirthing to your baby may be even greater than the experience of a calm and more comfortable birth for you.

*Katharine Graves*

# Foreword

This excellent hypnobirthing book will reach softly into the hearts and minds of parents approaching birth and fill them with inspirational visions of possibilities and aspirations for beautiful, peaceful, calm births for their babies and for themselves. Katharine's personal qualities – unfailing positivity, humour, the deepest respect for birth and for women, their partners and their babies, and a deep faith in the natural birth process – shine out of the pages of this splendid book.

As a midwife, I provide care to women throughout pregnancy, birth and beyond. Part of the midwife's role is to provide sound evidence-based information for couples about the various available options around birth and the many interventions in the physiological process which have become so routine that they are rarely questioned and, indeed, are widely believed to be true, despite, in some cases, an unsatisfactory or absent evidence base. The midwife then helps the couple to explore the risks and benefits of each intervention and the risks and benefits of declining these interventions, so that they can make an informed plan of their preferences.

Birth, of course, has its own agenda and does not always play out the way we might wish. Hypnobirthing is so important here too, as a calm mother can help her baby even during a complex or challenging birth. As a midwife, I also have a responsibility to inform the woman and her partner about their legal and moral rights in relation to accepting or declining aspects of health care offered to them.

Couples who are empowered by attending Katharine's KGHypnobirthing courses, and by reading this book, will be in a much stronger position to face this daunting task of making informed plans for pregnancy, birth and new parenting that are right for their family.

In this inspiring book, Katharine's philosophy challenges the widespread and insidious tocophobia (pathological fear of birth) which makes pregnancy and birth so challenging today. It will be an excellent additional resource in the long journey our society needs to take back towards embracing normal birth sensations.

KGHypnobirthing can, and frequently does, provide a way for a mother and her baby to have a calm, drug-free, gentle and more comfortable birth. Using hypnobirthing techniques, mothers are more in tune with their powerful inner strength and can experience the transformational nature of birth, emerging full of wonder at their new-found exhilaration and sense of their own power. Their babies are born smoothly and simply, requiring fewer of the interventions and medications that can make birth so hazardous for some. Their partners are in tune with the vital work of birth, ready to nurture and protect the mother as she births her child and to receive the baby with joy and love, drawing the new family into embracing and protective arms.

Peace on Earth begins with Birth.

Liz Nightingale
Midwife and KGH teacher
www.nightingalebirthfriend.co.uk

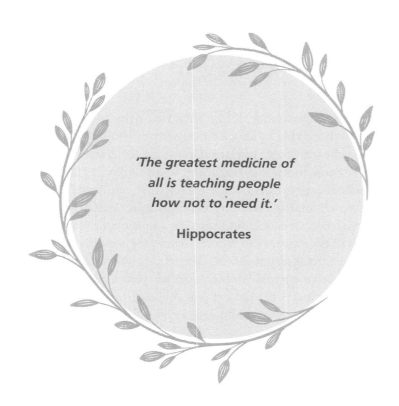

*'The greatest medicine of all is teaching people how not to need it.'*

**Hippocrates**

# CHAPTER 1

# KGHypnobirthing Explained

First it is important to define what I mean by 'hypnobirthing' and what is special about KGHypnobirthing. One woman may say she has done hypnobirthing, and maintains it didn't work – when all she did was listen to an audio during labour. It is plainly a great deal more effective if you have read this book which will make a big difference. Reading this book, doing the practice, and listening to a relaxation audio every day will make a great difference to your experience of giving birth, but you will get the full benefit if you attend a KGH face-to-face or virtual (zoom) course with a teacher (kghb. org/kghcourse). If this is not possible, you can purchase the KGH online course at kghb.org/kgh-online.

Doing the KGH course is a little like learning to play a musical instrument. I could tell you how to play the piano in ten minutes, but it wouldn't mean you could do it. If you went to lessons, you would progress. But if you practised between the lessons, you would progress much faster. KGH is made up of a lot of simple little things, because you can't be doing with complicated things when you're giving birth, but put together they make a very big difference. The more you practise, the better the outcome.

If you decide to enrol on a KGH course as a result of reading this book, please make sure it is the full 12-hour KGH course. Anyone can use the word 'hypnobirthing' attached to courses of different lengths and quality, so make sure you have reached the right place when you book.

Most women come to a KGH class with their partners; some come on their own. You can do it either way. Fathers often come to the class unwillingly, but by the end are the most enthusiastic advocates of the method and are so glad they came because they now have knowledge and a role at the birth. You may be surprised at the depth of knowledge you receive and also that the course is soundly based on evidence and logic.

KGH teaches a woman to work with her body, which is naturally designed to give birth. It releases the fear and negativity that she has been programmed with from an early age (everyone knows that birth is painful, don't they?), and replaces it with calm confidence. A mother who comes to the KGH class will often say that giving birth was the most wonderful and empowering experience of her life. That may be difficult for you to believe, but it is true. The reason you are reading this book is because that's how you would like your birth to be, and that's how it really can be. Yes, really.

As you read this book, you will probably see a great deal of sense in what I say. But you may come up against some ideas that you think are not for you and these suggestions could be the most important. If this happens, I would ask you very seriously to take a careful look at the things you DON'T like. Do some research and find out the facts. Think about it quietly. Look at the matter again with an open mind. Reconsider it in the light of evidence and the new information you now have. I'm not saying that I'm right and you're wrong. That would be presumptuous and impossible because I don't know your background and life story, but many so called 'decisions' are in truth assumptions: 'Everyone knows that', or, 'My friend says ... ' One of the biggest assumptions that people make is that it is safer to give birth in hospital than at home, in spite of the fact that the evidence tells us that homebirth is safer for a normal healthy woman. I'm simply suggesting that everything is important and, if you feel you want to reject something, it may be that it makes you feel uncomfortable because it conflicts with an assumption you have made or a preconception you have. Once you have done your research and reconsidered the question, if you decide to change your mind, that's fine. If you decide your original judgement was right, that's fine too. But you will be coming to a true decision from a place of knowledge, and not from a preconception based on nothing more than society's assumptions about birth.

I can promise you one thing about KGH, and that is that it will not be as you expect. Inevitably we approach people and experiences with an idea of what they are going to be like. The actual experience is always different, and that applies to this book and the KGH course too.

## The 'Hypno' word

Some people have used hypnotherapy very effectively to help them stop smoking or cope with a fear of flying, but for many people it is a word that conjures up images of stage hypnotists apparently making people cluck like a chicken or bark like a dog, or eat an onion thinking it's an apple. In fact, hypnotherapy is merely the use of words: words used in a more focused and positive way to help people let go of some of the negative ideas they have acquired in life. When you stop to think for a moment, our world view as an adult is simply the sum total of all the phrases we have heard and all the experiences we have had throughout our life; many of them are positive, but a few are negative.

For example, babies aren't born with a fear of spiders. They probably find the little wriggly creature quite interesting.

They learn fear from mum when she screams at the sight of a spider. If that child grows up with extreme arachnophobia and goes to a hypnotherapist for help, you could almost say they need to be un-hypnotised as the hypnosis, the mind changing, happened when the problem first arose. So in fact a hypnotherapist un-hypnotises people, which sounds much more user-friendly, and is actually true.

People's response to hypnotherapy is interesting too. I remember I was once working with a lady on weight loss and at the end of the session she said, 'It can't possibly have worked, because I heard every word you said, and I spent the whole time worrying that I hadn't turned off my phone and that it might ring.' Her perception was that, in hypnotherapy, you go into some curious, spaced-out state, and then words waft over you and a change happens. The funny thing is that she came back the next week and said, 'It was really strange, I just didn't want to pick at food during the week.' Plainly her conscious mind had been so busy thinking about her phone that the suggestions I had given had slipped in under the radar and had worked well.

On the other hand, someone else can be so relaxed that they are practically out for the count. They look as if they are asleep, but they are not, and they may well say, 'It can't possibly have worked because I didn't hear a word you said.' Their assumption is that, in order for anything to happen, the conscious mind has to think about it and process it. But hypnotherapy will work equally well for that person too. And you know they have heard because, at the end of the session, when you suggest they open their eyes and 'come back into the room', they do. So even though they appear to be asleep, something is still listening.

It is very interesting. It is simple, gentle and profound, and the person concerned is always in control.

## The power of language

Kipling said: 'Words are the most powerful drug known to man' – a pretty accurate statement, and he was right. A word in the right or the wrong place can make or ruin a friendship for life. When I remarked to a friend that I was going skiing, he said. 'Oh, do you still ski?' Now, 'Do you ski?' is a neutral question. 'Do you still ski?' means that you look so old and decrepit that I didn't think you could possibly stagger onto a couple of planks and slide down a mountain. I was very polite and I didn't laugh, because, if my friend had realised what he had said, he would have been mortified. But the word 'still' revealed exactly what he was thinking, and one little word made all the difference.

Similarly, women who were at home looking after a baby or a child used to be asked, 'Do you work, or are you just a housewife?' Now the first question, 'Do you work?' is insulting enough, and the only answer must be, 'I work 24/7. What are your hours?' But the second phrase is devastating. The little word 'just' turns you from a normal human being of average height and reasonable intelligence into something about 2cm high, without a brain, that someone could trip over without noticing. A comment like that can destroy your self-respect. In fact, because of the word 'just' that was so often associated with it, the word 'housewife' has almost become an insult and has dropped out of our vocabulary. People nowadays will use the phrase 'full-time mum', 'stay-at-home dad' or 'home-maker' instead.

We will look at more words as we go through, and please always be alert for those little words that can slip by un-noticed but tell you a great deal. " 'Just' hop up on the couch and I'll do your sweep now." " 'Just' a little cut," (for an episiotomy). They often mean that the person wants to play down what they are about to do and it is more significant than they want you to think. Notice, stop and think, before you make YOUR choice.

Words are very important, but they are even more important to a woman who is giving birth because the female of any species, including us, is at her most alert when she is giving birth because she is simultaneously at her most vulnerable. There could be a smell that attracts a predator, or it could be harder for her to run away if a predator appears, so she will naturally be many times more alert than in the normal course of events to protect the precious little bundle that she is about to produce. Therefore, she will be more aware of the tiniest little thing that could make her nervous or cause her stress.

I would like you to do a simple little exercise now. Put yourself into this extra state of alertness and be aware of the tiniest little changes in your mind or in your body and then ask yourself, 'Am I in pain?' Did the thought of pain enter your head when it hadn't been there before? Did you do a quick check to see if there was any discomfort in your body? Did you perhaps notice the slightest tightening of your forehead or your jaw?

Now settle yourself comfortably in the same alert way again and ask yourself, 'Am I comfortable?' Maybe the experience was different this time. Perhaps you felt your shoulders drop a little as any tension melted away?

So, if a midwife comes into the room when you are in labour and asks about pain, it is the role of the partner, their important protective role, to ask her not to use the word 'pain', explaining that words are important to you and have an effect. It is part of the partner's role as protector, to make sure the mother feels she is in a calm, safe space as she gives birth, and I'll explain why later on. 'Pain' is a perfectly good word in normal conversation, and the fact that everyone tells you that birth is painful (even though it doesn't need to be as we will see) is probably the reason why you are reading this book, but in labour it is actively harmful. It can make the mother think about having pain when she was not even considering it before; it can cause tension, and set her on a path of it becoming a self-fulfilling prophecy. It could even add a considerable time onto the length of labour. Labour is a very big event; it is also a very subtle event. One of the most important things that KGH birth partners do is to make sure the birthing woman feels calm and safe. I don't just mean with low lights and soft music but, more importantly, feeling calm mentally and emotionally.

A mother sent me this email which is an excellent example of the careless use of words:

> *'My husband and I participated in your KGH course and we both found it incredibly useful and inspiring. Since then we have been practising lots.*
>
> *I am now 39 and a half weeks pregnant and attended a midwife appointment this morning. She told me that my baby was in the 'wrong position', as the baby's back is against my back, and that I would therefore have a 'long and painful labour'. She said that I'm still allowed to go ahead with my homebirth, but that it is now likely that I will have to be transferred to hospital for an assisted delivery.*
>
> *As you can imagine this has got me into a right panic! I am now really worried about the birth (I had previously been looking forward to it) and frightened that I won't be able to cope. I've looked up exercises that I can do to help the baby move into a better position, but I would be incredibly grateful if you could suggest anything else to help with this situation.'*

Tell a mother that her baby is in the 'wrong position' and you can't do more to worry and upset her. The word *wrong*

– *wrong* – *wrong* is resonating in her subconscious mind – 'There's something wrong with my baby.' Add to this that labour will be 'long and painful' coming from someone with knowledge and experience. It could easily become a self-fulfilling prophecy. Then the words 'I'm still allowed' tell her that she is not sufficiently intelligent to make her own decisions but has to do what she's told like a small child. Next she is told that she will probably have to 'be transferred' – not that 'she will transfer', i.e. something she does, but that 'she will be transferred', i.e. it will be done to her. Then she is frightened by the prospect of an assisted delivery, forceps or ventouse (vacuum extraction), when she had been planning a natural birth. What more could you say in two sentences to terrify a woman about to give birth?

We did some work and restored her calm and confidence, and ten days later I received another email with her birth report:

*'I just wanted to let you know that we had our baby on Wednesday morning. A little girl.*

*Possibly due to the baby lying back to back, I felt the discomfort exclusively in my back, which led to the midwife on the phone initially telling me that I was not in labour. So, to cut a long story short, by the time a midwife came out to me three hours later I was already 7cm dilated … and I ended up having my baby in the birthing pool approximately seven hours after we made that first telephone call.*

*My waters didn't break at all, which I think must have helped the baby turn right at the last minute, just before she came out. So I think you were right when you said that "baby knows best".*

*Your support was absolutely invaluable during the run-up to the birth.'*

We will talk about a back-to-back baby in more detail later in the book. Here we are discussing the use of words. But sensations of a back-to-back labour are more likely to be experienced in the back, and the mother talks about discomfort but not pain. Midwives are sometimes fooled by how calm a KGH mother is, and don't realise how far her labour has progressed. Because the midwife on the phone didn't realise, the mother was able to labour undisturbed, so labour progressed well and she was 7cm dilated when the midwives arrived three hours later; 7cm in three hours is excellent progress for a first baby, regardless of which way it is facing. A labour of seven hours is also good for a first baby. Also, most back-to-back babies turn in labour, and it would have been consoling for the mother if the first midwife had told her this.

This story is a classic example of the harm careless words can do, and the difference words can make. I included it in the book as a particularly bad example, but a mother reported to me just recently that the same words had been used almost verbatim to her.

Because words are so powerful, we at KGH use them in a slightly different way. The word 'contraction' is made up of hard sounds: a 'c', 't' and 'n'. It is medical jargon, with connotations of pain. So we use the word 'surge' instead. It is made up of soft sounds that have a different effect. It conjures up images of the waves of the sea. Everything in nature works in that wavelike movement: the sea, light waves, sound waves, the rhythms of the seasons of the year and day and night all move in that wave-like movement, and certainly the muscles of the uterus in labour do. They start to work, build up to a peak, and release again. So not only does the word 'surge' have a more calming effect, but it is perhaps a more accurate description of what is going on. If English is not your mother tongue, there will certainly be a word in your own language that also has a soft sound that you can use.

You may feel rather silly and affected when you start to use the word 'surge' instead of 'contraction', but please persist. After a couple of weeks, it will feel quite normal. For a few people, the word 'wave' or 'rush' may be right for you, but give yourself a reasonable length of time to become accustomed to the word 'surge' first as I hope you can now see the reason why we ask you to do this.

You will see that all the small changes you learn about in this book put together make a very big difference.

Opposite is a table of some words and phrases that can cause stress and harm, with more positive replacements.

## The power of thoughts

Just as you will have a better birth experience if you use more positive words, so you will have an even more positive birth experience if you entertain more positive thoughts. Here is what you do to achieve this. Start by noticing the thoughts that come into your mind just as you are now beginning to notice the words you use. You might like to sit quietly for a few minutes to practise this, or you can allow it to happen as you go about your daily life. Just as you are starting to notice the words you use, so you are now starting to notice the thoughts in your mind. Once you are used to this, when you notice a negative thought entering your mind, just notice it drifting away. It can travel on a soft fluffy cloud if you find this helpful, or you can blow gently to help it on its way. Do it now. It feels good, doesn't it?

As you go through this book you will be given useful positive images and thoughts to put into your mind, and practice will reinforce them until they become second nature. This will be

## POSITIVE BIRTHING WORDS

| | |
|---|---|
| Delivery | Birth |
| Deliver | Give birth |
| Labour stalls | Take a rest for a while |
| Failure to progress | Labour is taking longer than expected |
| Pain | Sensation |
| High risk | May need extra help |
| Low risk | Normal and healthy |
| Contraction | Surge |
| Relax | Release, soften |
| Try | Creates stress and pre-supposes failure |
| What is your due date? | How many weeks pregnant are you? |
| Overdue/late | For what? |
| Just/only | It may be more significant than someone would have you believe. |
| Allow | It is you that does the allowing not your caregivers. It is you that chooses whether to allow someone to do something to you. |
| Outside guidelines | Implies that it is a dangerous or impossible course of action. Guidelines are to remind a health professional what they should offer to the woman. A woman then makes her choice whether to accept the offer. |
| Should, must | The guidelines say that any procedure is 'offered'. It is your choice whether to accept that offer. |
| Could happen | How likely is it to happen? |
| Risk averse | Pro medicalisation |

explained more fully later on, and it really makes a difference. When talking about how the mind works, the analogy has been used that the mind is like an iceberg. The conscious mind, the neocortex, is like the part you can see above the surface of the water. It is large and powerful and should be treated with great respect, and we are hugely privileged to have this amazing tool. But underneath the water is the far larger, and far more powerful, part of the iceberg, and this part is like the unconscious mind. It is difficult to answer questions about the unconscious mind because those questions come from the conscious mind – the thinking part of the brain, the part above the surface. The conscious mind can never really comprehend the unconscious mind. The unconscious mind is far larger, far more powerful, and should be treated with even greater respect.

A famous quote that is attributed to Einstein is: 'The intuitive mind is a sacred gift and the rational mind is a faithful servant. We have created a society that honours the servant and has forgotten the gift.' We are so busy thinking and working things out in our society, that we sometimes forget we have this more intuitive part of the mind.

The conscious mind is an amazing tool. Use it to find out the facts and make logical decisions in preparation for the birth of your baby. Look at the facts and the evidence when you are planning your birth. Choose the experts you want to work with. Make your choices based on evidence. You might take a year to plan your wedding so it is just as you had always dreamed. How much more important is the birth of your baby? It is the most important day in your baby's life, and one of the most important days in yours. You may engage an experienced wedding organiser, but you don't leave it to them to decide where the ceremony is to take place. You do your research, using their experience to help you, and make your choice. You don't arrive at the ceremony and hope the flowers, however beautifully arranged, will match the bridesmaid's dresses. You specify what you want so everything goes smoothly on the day.

It is the same with an athlete. They don't turn up at the stadium and hope to win a gold medal. The work is done in the weeks, months and years of training. They work with the carefully chosen team around them, the trainer, physiotherapist, massage therapist, PR person, psychotherapist or hypnotherapist, expert on kit, admin person, dietician, driver. All these people help them prepare, but they don't tell them what to do during the race. They check different styles of running, different pieces of equipment, different strategies. The runner runs the race on their own, and their team are in the background just in case they are needed, their work has already been done. Your gold medal at the end of your race is your baby.

The process of preparation is logical and well researched. The runner doesn't decide on a strategy because they feel more comfortable with it, they look at the evidence and the times on the stopwatch. The preparation time is the time to use the rational brain. Having set everything up for the best possible outcome, they can then rely on their instinct during the race itself to respond to the situation at the time. A woman's instinct should be treated with the utmost respect during the birth process, and she can trust it herself. Feeling and instinct are different. Of course you can still perform basic checks to make sure that mother and baby are well, but we will look at how amazing the system is that nature has put in place.

We need both parts of the mind. Use the faithful servant to prepare for birth and trust the sacred gift for the birth itself. We see it in animals: anyone who has a pet dog will know that it will probably be sitting on the doormat a few minutes before its owner comes home. The animal somehow knows, and we wonder at it.

But we have these instincts too. We have all had the experience of reaching out a hand to pick up the phone to call someone, maybe someone on the other side of the world to whom we haven't spoken for a couple of years, and just as we reach out, the phone rings and it's that person calling us. It feels so strange when this happens, because we don't understand it, but we've all had that experience and it's an example of the intuitive mind. Maybe that's how life really works.

## Negative thoughts

In the normal course of life, the words we hear go into our conscious mind are then processed by the unconscious mind, and have an effect right down to a cellular level of our bodies. We all know that, if someone says something that embarrassed us, we blush. If someone says something that is funny, we laugh.

So while you are pregnant it is very important that the input into your mind is positive. When pregnant women have been under stress – extreme stress, not just the normal ups and downs of daily life – their babies have not developed so well. Stress in the mother affects the baby from as early as 17 weeks, so it is important to maintain a positive environment and mindset. Sadly our current maternity services can subject a woman to a great deal of stress with the emphasis on risk and careless use of words. We will look at this in more depth a little later on but, between now and when your baby is born, avoid negative input, either thoughts, words or images. For instance, for the rest of your pregnancy, you are in charge of your television's remote control and the movies you stream. There is plenty to watch that is positive, funny, educational and light-hearted, and you and your partner can put off watching horror movies until after your baby is born.

As soon as you became pregnant, you probably found yourself beset by people telling you horror stories about birth. Why do people do this? Either because they think you are being naive when you talk about having a natural birth, but their opinion is not valid because they know nothing about KGHypnobirthing. Or it is cathartic for them because they have had a bad birth experience. Sadly that is the experience of many women, but it is not your role as a pregnant woman to provide catharsis for women who have had a bad experience.

This is actively harmful to you and to your baby, and no-one has the right to harm you in this way. We have been brought up to be polite and listen to what people say before we reply, but in this case please stop them. One mother used to say, 'I'm sorry, I can't be part of this conversation until after my baby is born, so could we have it then?'

Focus on where you want to be. You get what you focus on. If you drive down the road and try to avoid the potholes, what happens? You drive straight into them. If you want to avoid the potholes, you need to know that they are there, but then you focus on the flat parts of the road in order to avoid them. It's exactly the same with everything else in life. I'm not suggesting you should be unrealistic. Inform yourself well before you decide anything, then, having made the decision, put the negatives out of your mind and focus on where you want to be. Trust your instinct. That way you are far more likely to achieve your goal.

The mind doesn't take in the negative form. What is the image that pops into your head if you hear the phrase, 'Don't think of a pink elephant'? You can't get the image of the elephant out of your mind. When we start to notice, it is amazing how often we talk and think in terms of the negative. 'I'm not very good at this.' 'Don't do that.' If we want our partner to bring something home from the shops, how often do we say, 'Don't forget the bread?' 'Don't ... forget the bread.' It's just like the pink elephant. Then they come home without the bread and we say, 'I asked you to buy some bread. You always forget!' but you didn't, you specifically told them to forget the bread, and they did exactly what you asked. If you really want them to bring home some bread, you will be far more likely to get it if you say, 'Remember the bread.' Start to notice how often you use the negative, and re-programme yourself to use the positive. It makes a difference, and your life will improve immeasurably.

One dad we taught managed building sites. He had terrible trouble trying to make sure that the men wore their hard hats. Every morning he was telling them not to forget their hats. The morning after he attended the KGH course he told them to REMEMBER their hats and was amazed and delighted to see them all walking out on site wearing their safety helmets. It works!

The thoughts you take in last thing at night have eight hours to go on being processed, so it is particularly important that you go to sleep with a calm mind and positive thoughts about birth. How many people check their messages before they go to bed? If there happens to be a negative one, you may have trouble getting to sleep because you are worrying; your sleep will be disturbed, and you will wake feeling less refreshed in the morning. That is why in the KGHypnobirthing course you are given an audio to listen to last thing at night with positive statements and images about birth. This will be explained later on too.

## How other mammals give birth

When it comes to birth, we could learn a great deal from our fellow mammals. The conscious brain has little to do with the actual process of giving birth. We can't decide when our babies will be born, and we can't decide how our labour will be, though we can do a lot in preparation which affects this, because the thoughts we put in the mind affect the body.

If you have a cat, and you lovingly prepare a nice cosy box with a blanket in it in a warm corner of the kitchen for her to have her kittens, what happens? One day you notice that you haven't seen your cat for a while, so you mount a search and find her under the bed, or outside in the shed, with eight little kittens. She went to a small, safe place on her own where she felt private, safe and unobserved. Not where you thought she ought to be.

If a farmer has his ewes lambing in a barn, he knows that the one who is about to give birth is the one that retires to the furthest corner and becomes very still. It's the nearest she can get in that environment to going to her small, safe place and get away from the herd. If he goes into the house to make a cup of tea, there is a birth explosion in his absence, because the ewes feel safer not being observed.

Now please don't think I'm advocating giving birth without medical support; I am certainly not. But I am saying that if we respect our natural instincts, the birth is more likely to go smoothly and naturally. The more experienced your midwife, the less she will do or say. This is why research shows that giving birth at home is safer for most women and their babies. In the wild, an animal will take herself away on her own to a place where she feels safe to give birth. If she's not sure, the whole process will stop, or even reverse, until she is sure she has found a safe place to have her baby.

We know that animals follow their instincts, but we sometimes forget how powerful our own instincts are too. We are so busy using our brains that we forget that, in certain circumstances, they have their limitations. We know that we feel safe in some places and not in others. You can go into a house and it feels entirely like home; you go into another house and you know you could never live there because it just doesn't feel right. Your body relaxes when you are at home in your own safe space: somewhere that you feel comfortable and happy.

If you speak to a midwife who has supported mothers giving birth at home, she will say it is amazing the number of times she has been with a woman who has given birth in the toilet or in the bathroom. It is simply because the mother has gone instinctively to her small, safe place where she is generally private and alone and can shut out the world, so it is a natural place for her to want to be when she is having her baby. If you had forgotten to lock the door, and someone barged into the room when you were on the toilet, the whole process would stop and your body would stop working. The toilet may be a room upstairs at the back of the house, where other people are a long way away and the hurly-burly of the world is shut out. The reason that labour so often slows down when a mother goes to hospital and she can be sent home again, even two or three times, is simply that the hospital is a strange place and she is being observed by strangers, quite apart from the transfer from home to hospital, with bright lights and the sound of car horns and sirens all the way.

I often wonder how many mothers who arrive at hospital only to be told that they are only 1cm dilated, they are much too early and should go back home, were actually 4 or 5cm dilated when they left home, and it is just the unnatural experience of travelling across town and going to a strange

## THE 7 'C'S OF KGH: A SYNOPSIS OF KGH IN A NUTSHELL

**CHOICE** A KGH couple will have learnt about the decisions they may be asked to make, the alternatives available to them, and the implications of those choices. How can you achieve the birth you want without this information? You may not be told about it anywhere else.

**CONTROL** Once you are in a position to make an informed choice, that puts you in control. The experience of birth can make a difference to the rest of your life and the whole of your baby's life.

**CONFIDENCE** When you are in control – something that every couple I teach says that they want – that gives you confidence and puts you in a much better place to be than in a state of worry and stress.

**CALM** When you feel confident, your mind is calm, so you produce the hormone of calm, oxytocin, and the hormones of comfort, endorphins. Oxytocin is the hormone that makes birth efficient, and endorphins are the hormones of comfort, so labour becomes more comfortable.

**COMFORT** Therefore, when your mind is calm, labour can become more comfortable. KGH gives you the tools to help you to achieve this.

**COMMUNICATION** In order to achieve all this, you need good communication with your caregivers.

**CONSENT** When you have learnt KGH, you will be in a position to give informed consent or informed refusal to any intervention proposed.

place that has caused the body to tense up so the whole process has reversed.

I have a very good midwife friend who tells me of an occasion when she was caring for a mother in hospital who was doing well and was 6cm dilated when she was examined. Shortly after the examination, the senior midwife bustled into the room to check what was going on, examined the mother again, and found she was 3cm dilated. It was the arrival of a stranger; a slight rush (which is stress) that caused the process to reverse. Nobody had been unpleasant, nobody had been unkind, but the body had just said, 'I'm not quite sure about this,' and the whole process had reversed.

To have the best possible birth experience, we would do well to copy the instincts of our fellow mammals when it comes to giving birth. The only exception is to also have an experienced and unobtrusive midwife present. I am not advocating free birth. For everything else we can trust our fellow mammals to know what works.

## Takeaways

✳ Hypnotherapy is a benign, gentle and effective therapy using words to help you let go of a negative mindset or problem that you have acquired due to a previous negative life experience.

✳ Understand the power of language. Words are powerful and have a profound effect on how birth unfolds. Notice the words you use and make sure you have positive input.

✳ Harness the power of thoughts. Practise noticing the thoughts in your mind. Allow negative thoughts to drift away and replace them with positive thoughts.

✳ What is KGH? KGH is a lot of little things that, put together, make a big difference. The more of these things you do, the better your birth experience will be. It always makes a difference.

# CHAPTER 2

# The Logic of Labour

A mother who had recently used hypnobirthing came into a class to tell the couples about her experience. Her baby was born in three hours with no drugs, pain or tearing. Asked, 'Was it painful?', she replied, 'I can honestly say it wasn't painful, but I was amazed at how powerful it was.' Painful and powerful are different. We know what it feels like to use our muscles powerfully, but that doesn't have to be painful.

Here is a useful way of considering comfort:

## PAIN ⟶ COMFORT

You could consider comfort as being a continuum and everyone is naturally somewhere on this line. Using KGH always (and that's a pretty outspoken thing to say) moves you a good way along the line towards comfort. For some people it moves them all the way. One of the most important things to help you attain comfort is the practice you do.

There are three important questions to ask yourself too:
**Who** is going to be with you when your baby is born?
**When** will the birth happen – are you going to leave it to your baby to decide when to be born?
**Where** is the safest place for your baby to be born that is most likely to give you and your baby the safest birth and the best possible birth experience?

These questions are often not given enough consideration, and we will return to them as we go through the book.

First, we need to consider the question of fear. This is the root cause of pain in birth for a normal healthy woman. It may be panic, fear, or just stress or worry, but these are all degrees of the same thing. The problem is that fear causes the body to tense up, and when the body tenses up, it no longer works well, which causes pain. This concept was first identified by an obstetrician, Grantly Dick-Read about a century ago. He attended a birth in the east London slums where the woman

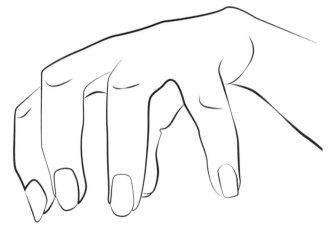

## THE FEAR/TENSION/PAIN CYCLE

Hold up your hand as if you are holding a tennis ball and tense your fingers. Can you move them? No. Now, with your hand in exactly the same position, relax your fingers. It's easy to move them now, isn't it? The same is true of the uterus. Can you see how labour would be long, and difficult, and painful because of the effect stress in your mind has on causing tension in your body?

declined pain relief and, when he enquired why, simply said, "It didn't hurt. It wasn't meant to, was it Doctor?" These simple words set him thinking, and it was he who came up with the fear/tension/pain cycle. This simple concept is the foundation of how the work of KGH has evolved a century later. Try doing the exercise opposite to demonstrate this.

## The uterus

Understanding how the hormones and the muscles of the uterus work is a very important part of KGH. Birth is an amazing and fascinating process.

The uterus is a powerful bag of muscles – possibly the strongest muscles in the body – which contains, protects and nourishes your baby. The powerful external vertical fibres of the upper part of the uterus work to draw up in a spiral motion in the first stage of labour. The powerful fibres of the middle layer of the uterus are interwoven with blood vessels and those of the inner layer form horizontal hoops around the cervix which, during pregnancy, keep your baby in. The deep muscles of the cervix at the neck of the womb need to be strong because they have a lot of weight to support when you are pregnant: the weight of the baby, the weight of the amniotic fluid, the pressure of the baby kicking, the pressure of you moving … they have an important job to do. In order for the baby to get out when it is ready, those strong muscles need to soften and move out of the way. We think of labour as the process of the baby moving out into the world, but most of labour is the process of the cervix softening, thinning and opening to facilitate the birth of your baby.

The higher, more superficial muscles of the uterus also need to support a lot of weight. They are assisted by the muscles of the abdomen, which are also very powerful.

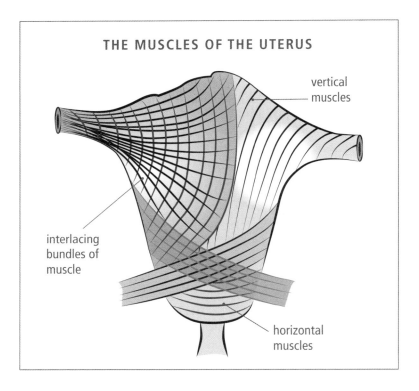

THE MUSCLES OF THE UTERUS

vertical
muscles

interlacing
bundles of
muscle

horizontal
muscles

During pregnancy, the body of the uterus must remain relaxed and able to stretch in order to accommodate the growing baby, while the cervix must remain firm in order to keep the baby in. In labour, these two functions are reversed. The muscles of the body of the uterus start to work and draw up, and the muscles of the cervix relax and start to open. The two types of muscle work in harmony, each with a different function, as long as the labouring woman is calm and relaxed as nature intended. In the first stage of labour, during surges, the vertical muscles draw up. The circular muscles relax and are drawn back in response. The cervix thins and opens. You can see the abdomen rising during a surge. I call it the 'up' stage of labour because that is what the muscles are doing.

When I was first told this I thought it was rather odd. How is it that two areas of muscle within the same organ, the uterus, respond in completely different ways to the same message which comes from the hormones and the nervous system? When I thought it through, I realised that actually it is perfectly logical because all the muscles in the body work in pairs. Some are a little more complicated, but the principle remains. If you want to do something as simple as bending your arm, the biceps muscle contracts and the triceps muscle releases. The triceps is almost redundant until you want to straighten your arm again, when the triceps works and the biceps releases.

So the different areas of muscle of the uterus function in exactly the same way as all the other muscles in the body, they work as a pair, which is just as well, because then you have a mechanism for getting back to normal afterwards. During birth, the upper muscles work and the deep hoops of muscle of the cervix release and after the birth the muscles of the cervix contract and the muscles further up release.

All the other muscles in the body are usually comfortable doing the job they are designed to do, but the only muscles that are generally considered to be painful are the muscles of the uterus, which seems an appallingly bad design fault when you consider that these are the muscles which ensure the continuation of the human race.

Bear in mind also the miracle that is the human body. It is miraculous how the body heals a cut. And yet these very important muscles of the uterus are generally considered to be uncomfortable, if not painful, when performing the function they are designed to do.

Let us consider what is happening. If you have pain in your muscles it is generally because you have undertaken some unusual and strenuous exercise. If you suddenly went for a

30km hike, the muscles in your legs would be painful the next day. If you painted all the ceilings in your home, your arm muscles would be stiff and sore the next day. But nobody ever had labour pains the next day, so this can't be the answer. Now imagine that you had painted all the ceilings in your home, and the next morning you went to lift a mug down from a shelf to make your morning coffee. The movement of your arm would probably be slow and inefficient and painful simply because, as the biceps muscle went to work, the triceps would be stiff from the previous day's activity and therefore would not be releasing so that, as you moved your arm, there would be a battle going on between the two muscles.

It is exactly the same with the muscles of the uterus: as the upper muscles of the uterus work to draw up, if the muscles of the cervix remain tense and do not release, there is a battle between the two sets of very powerful muscles. This means that each surge is more uncomfortable, less efficient and longer, there are more of them, and labour is longer.

Not only that but, because the muscles are working against each other, they tend to restrict the mother's blood supply. Blood carries oxygen, the primary fuel for each cell in the body, as well as nutrients. For muscle cells to work well they need a good supply of oxygen so, if the oxygen supply to the muscles is restricted, they will work less efficiently. If an athlete's muscles are deprived of oxygen they collapse with cramp. In addition, the oxygen carried in the mother's blood is the oxygen which goes through the placenta to the baby, so the baby's oxygen supply can be compromised. Therefore the baby is more likely to be in distress, so everything is progressing less than optimally.

On the other hand, as the upper muscles of the uterus work to draw up, if the muscles of the cervix gently release with each surge, then each surge is more comfortable, more efficient and shorter, there are fewer of them and labour is shorter.

It's very, very simple, and very, very logical.

## The emergency response – the sympathetic nervous system

Then we need to ask the question, 'What tips the mother from the relaxed response to the tense response?' And the answer is: fear. This is how we are designed to deal with emergencies. We call it the sympathetic nervous system. It is a brilliant system that evolved many millennia ago to act as a lifesaver in emergencies, and it works well. But the emergencies we met then were different from the emergencies we meet now. Thousands of years ago you might have been wandering over the brow of a hill and seen a sabre-toothed tiger in the valley in front of you. So what would you do? You'd freeze – and hope you hadn't been seen! If you had been seen you'd run, and if you couldn't run fast enough only then would you turn and fight. We tend to call it the fight–flight response, but actually it's the freeze–flight–fight response in that order. We all still have it, and it is how we deal with emergencies. The freeze–flight–fight response works in all of us.

The part of this response that is relevant to a woman in labour is the freeze response, because she is not going to be running or fighting. It is the rabbit in the headlights phenomenon. It is what happens when you are in a meeting and someone puts you on the spot by asking a difficult question, and you simply can't think of the answer, even though you are aware that you know it perfectly well. It can happen in an exam, in an interview, or just in a normal conversation too. And the moment you get home the answer comes back to you, and you say to yourself, 'Why couldn't I have thought of that earlier?' If you play a musical instrument, it's quite likely that your fingers will begin to stumble if someone comes into the room – you're being observed so you tense up and it's sufficient to disturb your hand–eye–brain coordination. That's the freeze response.

The minute you're put under stress, both the mind and the body freeze. If a mother feels afraid, or even slightly worried or nervous (it doesn't have to be abject terror; it can be quite a minor stress), her body freezes and labour slows down or stops. Labour is an important event, it is also a very subtle and nuanced event. How often is the cascade of medical interventions started by a stalled labour or a labour that fails to start at all? And what is often the reason for this? Stress, or worry. The human race has survived for millennia because it is a mother's instinct to protect her child, and part of this instinct programmes her to be in a small dark place, hidden away, where she feels absolutely safe before her body is prepared to release her baby and give birth. If she feels under the tiniest and most subtle of stresses, the body simply doesn't work, and yet our maternity system heaps progressively more stress on women from 40 weeks of pregnancy, and often before. I am not advocating giving birth alone without medical support, but it has been observed that a quiet birth with a known carer in a known environment frequently progresses well.

Continuity of care from a known carer reduces miscarriage by 19 per cent, pre-term birth by 24 per cent, and losing a baby in the first month by 16 per cent. It reduces the use of an epidural, an episiotomy, forceps or ventouse, induction of labour, and pain. There is a higher chance of a spontaneous vaginal birth, with shorter labour. Women report greater satisfaction in their birth experience, so there is a lower incidence of postnatal depression. Some people say that the best environment for giving birth is similar to the best environment for a natural conception: low lights, soft music, privacy, gentle stroking and plenty of time.

No animal will leave a trace of itself in a strange place if it can possibly help it; there might be a predator around. We know this in practice too. If you go away for a weekend, maybe staying in a beautiful place, very often you will be just a little bit constipated, and the body will not release until you are home again. Or you can be coming home from work, by car or walking down the road, thinking of this and that, and the minute you enter your own front door you need a pee. It's simply due to a natural mental and physical relaxation from being in your home: your own safe place. A baby is a very large and important part of ourselves. How much more careful will a mother's body be in choosing where she expels her baby compared with where she is prepared to expel her normal bodily excretions? It is our instinct to protect our young from predators. In labour, the female of any species is at her most vulnerable. There might be a smell that attracts a predator, and she's at her most immobile so she can't run away.

So when a mother feels stressed or fearful, what happens? The hormones she produces are affected. The hormones of pregnancy, labour and birth are a miraculous cocktail and a very complex subject. So let's take a simple look at this. When we are in the emergency response – when the sympathetic nervous system is activated – we produce hormones called catecholamines and in particular adrenaline, which is the most relevant hormone from our point of view.

We all know what an adrenaline rush feels like. Maybe you have been driving down a road when a car shoots out in front of you. You jam your foot on the brake and it feels almost like an electric shock shooting down your back. Your heart starts to thump, pumping blood around your body in case you need to run or fight. And your eyes are out on stalks panning to surrounding area for predators, because if there has been one sabre-toothed tiger there might be another. The same thing happens when you hear a sudden loud noise that makes you jump.

All your resources, all your energy, go to your arms and your legs, ready to run or fight – which is a great system for dealing with sabre-toothed tigers but absolutely useless when you're in labour, because you are not going anywhere.

## TESTING THE SYMPATHETIC NERVOUS SYSTEM

Stand up and hold one arm straight up in the air beside you and the other down at your side. Now open and close your fists very quickly. Keep going for a few minutes.

Do your arms feel the same? You probably found that the arm held above your head is beginning to ache, and the longer you continue the more painful it becomes and the arm down by your side is still perfectly comfortable. Bring the arm that you were holding up in the air down now, and notice how long it takes for that sensation to fade.

So what happened? The blood was draining away from the arm above your head and lactic acid was building up. It didn't take many minutes for this to happen, but it took quite some time for the feeling to fade away. Your upper and lower arms were both working in the same way; however, the blood supply was reaching your lower arm, but not your upper arm.

It is similar when we are in the emergency response in labour and the blood supply flows to the arms and the legs ready to run or fight, and away from those powerful uterine muscles which need a good blood supply in order to work effectively and comfortably. No wonder labour becomes painful if a woman is stressed or worried. This shows why the work we do to build positivity and confidence is so important.

That's how the sympathetic nervous system works. When you are in labour, the muscles of your uterus are working very powerfully for one minute, and remember powerful muscles need a good blood supply. What's more, in established labour, there are only two or three minutes in between surges, so there is not sufficient time for recovery. Remember: even elite athletes collapse with cramp if their muscles don't have a good blood supply.

## The calm normal situation – the parasympathetic nervous system

The other system that controls our responses is the parasympathetic nervous system. This is the state we are in most of the time because fortunately most of the time is not an emergency. It's the calm, normal response. The two systems cannot function at the same time. It's either one or the other. It's rather like standing half way up the stairs. You can't go up and down at the same time. You may be feeling confident and at ease as you read this book, so your parasympathetic nervous system is functioning, and you feel confident and relaxed.

When we are in the confident response – when the parasympathetic nervous system is activated – we produce the hormone oxytocin (again looking somewhat simplistically at this complex system). Oxytocin has been described by the Swedish scientist Kerstin Uvnäs-Moberg as the hormone of 'calmness and co-operation'. Michel Odent, the French natural birth pioneer, calls it the hormone of love, because we produce great peaks of it at special times in our lives: when we fall in love and when we make love, and the biggest peak of all is the one a mother produces just after she has given birth. It promotes the bonding of mother and baby and the establishment of breastfeeding. Oxytocin is less likely to be produced when we feel observed, so it has also been described as the 'shy hormone'. It makes us like privacy; we don't feel quite so relaxed in the company of strangers.

We love the feeling oxytocin gives us; we are addicted to it and would do practically anything for a fix. It is probably the hormone that has ensured the continuation of the human race. Oxytocin is also the hormone that makes the uterine muscles work in labour as there are oxytocin receptors in the uterus. As long as you are feeling confident, calm and harmonious, you will naturally produce this hormone, which makes the uterine muscles work and makes labour efficient.

Other important hormones we produce in the parasympathetic nervous system, or the confidence response, are endorphins. Endorphins, as their full name 'endogenous morphine' (morphine produced in the body) implies, are related to morphine. Morphine is the most powerful artificial pain-relieving drug that we have. We give it to people after major surgery and with advanced cancer. Endorphins, which we produce naturally in our own bodies, have been said to be many times more powerful than morphine. In her book *The Oxytocin Factor*, Kerstin Uvnäs-Moberg says that when we feel calm and confident, the elevated level of oxytocin in the body seems to result in the increased secretion of endorphins. So if the mind is in the right place, the body naturally produces oxytocin to make labour efficient, and endorphins to make it comfortable.

When a mother is in the parasympathetic nervous system, all her resources, her blood supply and oxygen, go to her internal organs – her digestive and reproductive organs. This is obviously a far more efficient use of resources when she is giving birth. She can digest food to keep her energy up, and the powerful muscles of the uterus need a good blood supply in order to work well. This is also the blood supply that carries oxygen and nutrients to the placenta for the baby. It is a much more effective use of energy than diverting it to the arms and legs, as with the fear/emergency response.

The system is perfect, and already in place. It is very simple: the most beautiful shining diamond of perfection.

The trouble is that we tend to get in the way, and hypnobirthing is the system that helps us to get out of the way of this perfect system and allow it to work well.

What is it that trips us from the parasympathetic nervous system, the confident response, to the sympathetic nervous system, the emergency response? It is two things – fear, stress or worry, and being observed or watched. It is why many people are petrified of public speaking. It is totally unnatural for any animal to stand out in the open and be observed. They skulk in the undergrowth, or seek safety in numbers in a herd, or they are camouflaged against their background like a camel in the desert. It's also why labour frequently slows down when a mother arrives at a birth centre or hospital. However carefully the environment is created to be homely, and however well-meaning the midwives, she is still in a strange place being observed by strange people, and the natural response of her body is to freeze. It doesn't have to be abject terror; it is simply a very subtle, animal suspicion. Instinctively she doesn't feel safe.

So the important thing that affects labour is what is happening in the mind. We know this is true, because every top sportsman, every top football team, has a sports psychologist. A player may have the right physique and do all the training and practice, but if their mind isn't in the right place they won't get to the very top of their sport. You could regard hypnobirthing as the sports psychology for giving birth!

## ACHIEVING CONFIDENCE OVER FEAR

You cannot be in both the sympathetic and the parasympathetic nervous systems at the same time. In other words, you cannot be in both the fear response and the confident response. Let's just recap what we have learned in this chapter.

The body is designed to produce oxytocin, which makes birth efficient, and endorphins, which make birth comfortable, as long as your mind is in a calm, safe and harmonious place. The system for a calm and comfortable labour is perfect; it is already in place.

All we need to do is let go of the fears, worries and negative thoughts that we have all acquired about birth, get out of the way and let the system work.

This is why KGH is so successful. Every time you practise the techniques you are letting go of the assumptions, the preconceptions, the stresses and the tensions. You are releasing – allowing your body to give birth more naturally, comfortably and easily.

# *Takeaways*

✳ The muscles of the uterus and the cervix work as a pair to facilitate birth.

✳ The body is perfectly designed to give birth efficiently and comfortably.

✳ The hormones that facilitate a comfortable birth or lead to a painful birth are controlled by our state of mind.

✳ If the mind is calm we create oxytocin to make labour efficient and endorphins to make it comfortable.

✳ The natural place to give birth is a small safe place with privacy.

✳ Continuity of care leads to better outcomes.

# CHAPTER 3

# The Mind/Body Effect and Breathing for Birth

The thoughts in your mind affect your body. If somebody is feeling down, you can instantly see it in the way they walk. If you have to tell someone bad news, you suggest that they sit down first in case they feel weak at the knees. If you tell someone something that embarrasses them, they blush. But we sometimes under-estimate just how powerful the mind is. We tend to assume that everything happens in the body, and that the mind merely has some effect on what goes on.

## The power of the mind

Let us now consider the power of the mind. When you think about it, the body is merely a hunk of meat. It does absolutely nothing without the mind telling it to. So effectively, everything happens in the mind, and the body just trots dutifully along behind and does what it is told.

I'd like you to do a little exercise with each other as a couple, or with a friend (see page 51 for an illustration).

Stand opposite each other, and mothers, put your hand palm upwards on your partner's shoulder. Make sure the palm is facing up, otherwise you can twist your elbow. Now partners, bend her arm downwards at the elbow and mothers, try to resist them with all your strength. Now, her arm will probably· bend, though you may be surprised how strong she is.

Just relax for a minute. Mothers, shake your arm out, then put your arm back right on top of their shoulder in a very relaxed way. This time remain relaxed, and focus your attention on the tips of your fingers or even beyond, maybe looking towards a picture on the wall, or out of the window. Or you could imagine that you are standing on a mountain looking at the view, or a similar distant view, perhaps looking out to sea. What can you see? A village in the valley? People? Cattle? Mountains? Boats? Islands? Waves? Tell your partner the details of what you see to keep your attention focused into the distance.

Now partners, try once more to bend her arm. Do it gently to start with because she has not done this exercise before. Help her to keep her attention right out in front of her, but build up the pressure on the arm gradually. Mothers, you may find that, as long as your focus stays out there, the arm is much stronger than it was before. It also feels much easier to hold the position of your arm than when you were resisting only with physical strength the first time. Interesting! Practise this a few times. As with everything, we get better with practice.

The Unbendable Arm Exercise shows us that if you relax and focus your attention, your body works better and more easily than when we use our physical strength alone.

Try this next exercise, the Lemon Tree Script (see page 53), too. You can download the music to play in the background from the website www.kghypnobirthing.com. The music I use for practice and as the background music to our audio is the gentle Armenian Lullaby. It is music played on a real piano by a real person, rather than electronic music, which has a completely different effect. A partner can read the script for mothers, and then swap over, so that you can both experience it.

## THE UNBENDABLE ARM EXERCISE

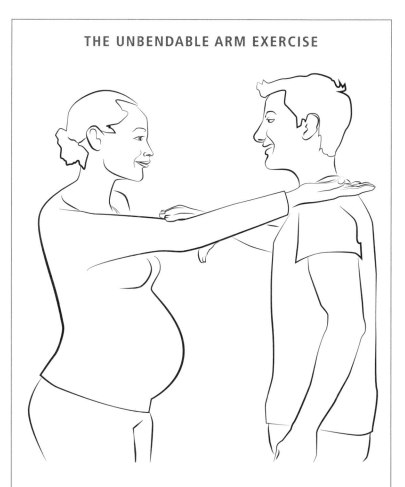

The Unbendable Arm Exercise is a really interesting demonstration of the power of the mind and how, when you can harness that power to work together with your body you become stronger and more powerful. In labour, this knowledge and practice will help your body to work better.

## THE LEMON TREE SCRIPT

Close your eyes, make yourself comfortable and relax.

Breathe in and out deeply three times, saying to yourself on the out breaths, 'Release', 'Soften', 'Comfort'.

Now just sit there for a few moments as you let your whole body and mind become calm and relaxed. Continue to breathe slowly, deeply and gently, as you feel your body becoming soft, weightless, totally comfortable.

Imagine yourself on a lovely warm summer's day sitting under the shade of a lemon tree. Beside you is a table which has on it a board and a knife, an empty glass, and a bottle of sparkling water chilled in an ice bucket. The scent of lemons is all around you, and each time you breathe in, the pleasant scent fills your nostrils.

You decide to make yourself a cooling and refreshing drink with a squeeze of fresh lemon in the sparkling water to quench your thirst. So you pick a lemon off the tree, and even as you do that your body begins to respond to the knowledge that soon it will be tasting a refreshing lemon drink.

You put the lemon on the board to cut it in half and, as you do that, lemon juice runs onto the board and onto your fingers, while the smell of lemon gets even more powerful in your nostrils.

Now you bring your fingers up to your mouth to lick them and, as your fingers approach your mouth and nose, the smell of lemon is very strong, and you start salivating even before your fingers reach your mouth.

Now you lick your fingers and your whole mouth fills with saliva from the tang of the lemon juice as your tongue washes lemon flavour all round your mouth.

As you sit relaxed, with your mind in that garden, with saliva filling your mouth with the taste of lemon juice, you realise that this is happening to you right now, in this very moment, as you understand that your mind produces sensations that your body acts upon.

And now you come back to the present with the memory and knowledge of how the mind and body act together so powerfully, and the knowledge that this mind/body relationship is an effective tool for you to use when you give birth to your baby. And now open your eyes and let the taste ebb away.

What happened then?

Many people find that they salivate. You may have, you may not have. If I tell you to salivate you can't do it on command; it's an involuntary response. But the ideas that you put in your head can make you salivate, just like Pavlov's dogs. It's just the same with labour. Labour is an involuntary response, but the ideas that you put in your head can affect its progress and its comfort.

Not everybody will salivate during the Lemon Tree exercise. Most people do, but a few don't because everybody is different – we all respond to different things and learn in different ways. For example, some people are visual learners, who learn from seeing how things are done, while others are more auditory and prefer to be talked through things. That's why you are given many different things to practise in hypnobirthing. You don't have to do them all, but simply choose those you like best.

This is good to know, because people sometimes have a fear that hypnotherapy can make you do or say something you would rather not – which is completely impossible, because nobody can use hypnotherapy to make you do something when you don't want to, or that is not in your best interests.

To re-cap these two exercises:

The first, the Unbendable Arm Exercise, shows that if you relax and focus your attention, your body works better and it's easier to do what you want to do.

The second, the Lemon Tree Script, shows that the thoughts you put in your mind affect the involuntary responses of your body.

Both these exercises prove that the practice we are going to do actually works, and will have a positive effect on labour and birth, so it's definitely worth doing.

## Up breathing

There are two types of breathing in KGH. The first we'll learn is the breathing to do during surges in the up (first) stage of labour. It is also the breathing you use during practice. Because the muscles are drawing up during a surge, I gave it the name 'up breathing', and it is very simple. It is a long, slow breath, in through the nose and out through the slightly open mouth.

The purpose of this breath is to use the absolute minimum of muscular effort, so that the muscle used in breathing, the diaphragm, in no way interferes with the working of the muscles of the uterus that are very close below by the end of pregnancy. We breathe in through the nose because it is a natural way of breathing; we breathe out through the slightly open mouth because that gives a feeling of release, of letting go, and that is exactly what we want to achieve. The out breath is naturally a little longer than the in breath, and it's on the out breath that we produce more oxytocin (Uvnäs-Moberg). Even something as simple as a few slow, deep breaths can help you feel more relaxed and completely change the atmosphere around you. Try that now and you'll see that it's true.

## UP-BREATHING IMAGES

This is a long, slow breath in through the nose and out through the mouth, focusing your attention upwards.

**As you breathe in,** watch the sun rise, the beautiful pink appearing on the horizon.

**As the sun rises,** so your body draws gently upwards.

**Breathe out** with the sun as it rises higher in the sky, and see the pinkness reflected on the clouds above.

**Breathe in,** and see yourself blowing bubbles, and see them get bigger and bigger.

**As you breathe out,** watch the bubbles float upwards into the sky, upwards into the sky, drawing upwards with each relaxing breath.

**Breathe in** and imagine yourself beside a huge, brightly coloured hot air balloon as it is being inflated.

**Breathing out,** just watch the balloon floating higher and higher into the sky until it's so high it looks tiny.

**Breathing in,** imagine a beautiful soft, velvety, full-blown rose.

**Breathing out,** bury your face in the rose and feel the velvety softness and smell the beautiful perfume.

**Breathing in,** watch a pebble drop into a pond and the ripples flow out.

**Breathing out,** the ripples flow wider, smoother, more open.

**Breathe slowly,** and very comfortably.

**With each soothing breath** your body becomes more relaxed and calm.

**Breathe up** as your mind and body work together in unison.

**You're doing really well;** that's very good.

**So calm,** so serene, so at peace.

If you're a flautist or a singer your breaths will naturally be longer. But the really important thing is that you're not straining to achieve a particular length of breath, and that it is entirely relaxed. Of course, as you practise it will become more natural and the breaths will gradually lengthen.

Your natural length of breath also depends upon the stage of pregnancy you are at because, as your baby grows, your lung capacity is gradually reduced. And then, in the last couple of weeks before birth, the baby's head engages in your pelvis, your baby moves down, and you can breathe more easily. This is why there is no suggested count to this breathing. If there were, you would aspire to reach it, and that would introduce tension.

Practise this now, breathing in slowly through the nose and releasing the air slowly through the slightly open mouth. Now do the same again, but this time do three breaths, because three or four breaths are more like the length of a surge.

We know that the uterine muscles are working to draw up, and we know that the mind is powerful and affects the body. We have just done exercises to prove it. Therefore, if the muscles of the body are working to draw upwards, you want the mind to be thinking 'up' so that mind and body are working together. So there are some visualisation images to go with this breathing on page 55. Also, the cervix, the neck of the womb, is softening and opening so we need soft and open images in the mind to facilitate this as well.

Practise the up breathing exercise with these images. It's ideal to have someone to talk you through the images, and they can use the suggestions on page 55, but you can practise on your own as well, and you will soon remember the images you need to visualise.

It's much easier to visualise with your eyes closed, so you are not distracted by whatever is going on around you. So, allow your eyes to gently close, and then on the next breath watch the sun rise, the beautiful pink appearing on the horizon, and as you breathe out, breathe up with the sun as it rises higher in the sky.

On the next breath, see yourself blowing bubbles, see them getting bigger and bigger, and as you breathe out watch the bubbles float away upwards into the sky. Take one more breath, and as you breathe in, notice that with each upward breath your body becomes more relaxed and calm, and as you exhale, breathe up as your mind and body work together in harmony.

Now breathe in and imagine you are standing beside a huge hot air balloon as it is inflated. See how big it is. See the bright colours. And as you breathe out, the tethers are released and it floats gently upwards until it's tiny, right up high in the sky.

Two effective soft and open images are:

As you breathe in, imagine a beautiful full-blown rose, soft, open, velvet, voluptuous. As you breathe out, bury your face in its petals, feel the velvety softness on your cheeks, smell the beautiful perfume. In another country it might be more appropriate to use a different flower such as a lotus flower.

Alternatively, watch a pebble drop into a pond and, as you breathe in, see the ripples go out and out and, as you breathe out, they go wider, more fluid, smoother, and more open.

These visualisation images may be helpful, but you can use anything that is comforting and relaxing for you and which has an 'up' or soft and open emphasis. You may find it helpful if your birth companion prompts you with these suggestions during surges. Partners are welcome to use their own words, but, if they have been up all night, they may not be at their most creative at 3am, so it can be useful to have some suggestions ready. Or they can say the same thing over and over again, which is quite soothing, like a mantra. And some women prefer silence.

Even something as simple as relaxed breathing gets better with practice. So I would suggest that you practise this slow breathing together with the images a couple of times a day. For many couples, the best times of the day can be first thing in the morning and last thing at night, because then you are most likely to be together. But if this is not your first baby, early morning is probably not a peaceful time, so it might be when you come home from work, or another time that works for you. Take just two or three minutes to practise the breathing using images just as you have done now, so that it becomes second nature.

The up breathing is what you will use during surges in the up stage of labour, and also for practising relaxations in pregnancy. It is useful at other times too, for example, before an antenatal visit, if you decide to go to a consultation with an obstetrician (your choice), before a vaginal examination, before someone takes a blood sample, at shift changes during labour, and other times too.

It is a very practical and useful life skill in your daily life. You might like to pause and take three of those lovely long, slow breaths, before you start work each day, when you come home from work, before a meal, before a job interview or doing a presentation. This will make a massive difference to your life experience

## Down breathing

The first type of breathing you have learnt above is for use as the muscles draw up in the first stage of labour, and the cervix thins and opens. As the muscles draw up, they gather at the top of the uterus ready to ease the baby out into the world. Yet again a brilliant system where everything works synergistically with everything else.

The second breathing we do, the 'down' breathing, is for use once the cervix is fully opened and the baby is moving down the birth canal into the world. It is a quick breath in through the nose, and a longer breath out through the nose.

The reason for breathing out through the nose this time is that it is a much more focused breathing, still relaxed but focused. It is almost as if your breath is following your baby down; you can practically feel it on the pelvic floor focusing downwards – not forcing downwards, but definitely focusing downwards. Try it for yourself a few times: a short breath in through the nose and a longer breath out through the nose, focusing your attention downwards. Practise a few breaths of the 'down' breathing now, taking a short breath in through the nose and releasing the air through a longer breath out through the nose.

Just like the up breathing, there are visualisation images to go with the down breathing; an image of anything that is gently downwards to facilitate the downward movement of your baby. We use the same soft and open images as with the up breathing mentioned previously. This time it is to facilitate the birth canal being soft and open as your baby passes out into the world.

A helpful image with a downward emphasis is of a little waterfall. If you were to go for a walk in the hills and find a stream trickling down into a small waterfall, you could sit there entranced for hours, watching the sunshine glinting on the drops of water.

If you're having your baby in the winter, you might like to imagine snowflakes dancing lightly downwards in beautiful patterns. Any soft and open or 'downwards' images like these are very helpful and effective.

## DOWN-BREATHING IMAGES

This is a short, quick breath, but still relaxed, in through the nose, and a longer breath out through the nose, focusing your attention downwards.

**Your body eases your baby** gently down with each breath.

**Imagine an entrancing waterfall**, with the water flowing gently downwards. Sunshine sparkling on the drops of water.

**Trust the gentle downward movement** of your body and your baby.

**Watch snowflakes dancing** lightly and gently downwards.

**Imagine the colours of the autumn leaves** as they float downwards.

**See the blossom**, pink and white, drifting down from a tree.

**Your baby moves** easily downwards.

**With each breath**, your baby is coming to you.

**Focus your attention** down towards your baby.

**You will soon** be holding your baby in your arms.

**Imagine a beautiful full-blown rose**, so soft and velvety and open.

**Watch the ripples** flowing out and out as a pebble drops into a pond. Fluid and smooth and open.

*'I can honestly say that hypnobirthing has changed my life. I use the breathing techniques daily to overcome any anxiety and am in awe of what my body can do by tuning in to the skills I have learnt.*

*Whilst I was pregnant, I also qualified as a KGHypnobirthing teacher, which further helped to compound my knowledge and understanding of its power, and, once I am ready, I hope to treach other couples in the future.'*

**Katy**

If your baby is likely to be born in autumn, leaves, yellow, gold, red, brown, floating downwards can be an excellent image and, for a summer baby, maybe you would like to bring to mind the pink and white blossom drifting downwards from a tree and making a carpet on the ground. Any gentle 'downwards' images like these are very helpful and effective.

You might again like to visualise the ripples going out as a pebble is dropped into a pond; the ripples flow out and out and out, so fluid and soft, smoother and smoother. It's a lovely visualisation.

Or it can be helpful to imagine a full-blown rose, or any flower you like. It feels so soft and velvety on your cheeks as you inhale its sweet fragrance. It is a soft and open image, and, if your mind is thinking soft and open, the birth canal is becoming soft and open. You may have seen a time lapse image of a flower opening, and imagining something like that can work well.

Your partner can read these visualisation prompts (page 60) to you while you practise the down breathing.

Take a few minutes to practise the down breathing with the downwards and soft and open and images. Take a quick breath in, and as you breathe out imagine that full-blown flower, beautiful, soft, velvety and voluptuous. Breathe in, and then breathing out see the ripples going out on the pond, fluid, soft and open. Once more, breathe in, and as you breathe out imagine that delightful little mountain waterfall. You can sit there entranced watching the sunshine on the drops of water, downwards, soft and gentle. This time, breathe in and imagine the snowflakes dancing gently and lightly downwards.

As with the images for the up breathing, keep it simple. For both stages I have given you lots of examples, but you might find that you prefer just to say the same thing over and over again, like a mantra. The phrases I have given are only suggestions, but at three in the morning when you're not at your best, they can be useful to have at hand. And if your partner is reading for you and you would find a different image more helpful, then they can change to something else. But, partners, you can say whatever you like, or keep it really simple. Saying something as simple as 'You're doing really well and I love you,' is more than adequate. Use the examples as guidelines which you may find useful during labour.

Please start practising the down breathing from about week 36 of your pregnancy. Have your partner read aloud so that you can practise the visualisations, and it all becomes intuitive ready for when your baby is born. Many women have said they couldn't have done it without their partner, and it was their partner's voice that carried them through.

Practise on the toilet as well. Sometimes in late pregnancy you can get a little constipated. After all, there is a head in your pelvis! Practising the down breathing on the toilet proves to you that it works even before you have your baby. It is multi-tasking – very efficient – and a useful life skill.

## *Takeaways*

* If you relax and focus your attention, your body works better, and the activity becomes easier. The Unbendable Arm Exercise can help you to really understand this.

* The thoughts you put in your mind affect even the involuntary response of your body. The Lemon Tree relaxation script is a useful demonstration.

* Up breathing using visualisation images helps your body to relax and work instinctively during surges in the up stage of labour. It has other applications too.

* Down Breathing using visualisations and images helps your baby to move downwards during the down stage of labour.

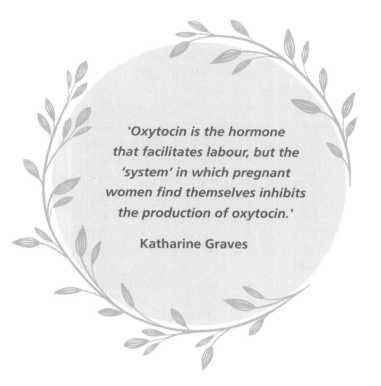

'Oxytocin is the hormone that facilitates labour, but the 'system' in which pregnant women find themselves inhibits the production of oxytocin.'

Katharine Graves

# CHAPTER 4

# Relaxation Practice

A note first of all about practice. You may think that you will read this book and apply the techniques in it when you give birth. No, that's not how it works. KGH is not done when you learn the techniques, it's not done at the birth, it's done in the practice between reading this book or attending your course with a KGH teacher and when you give birth. This is very important, and all the good birth reports I receive tell me that the couple practised lots.

It's just the same with everything else in life. You spend a long time planning a holiday, thinking of which country you would like to visit, where you would like to stay, when you would like to go. You don't just get into a car with an unknown driver, however skilled, and hope they will take you where you want to go. You don't just get onto a plane and hope it is going to your destination of choice. If you are going skiing you might do some exercises to get fit or have a few runs on a dry ski slope as well.

If you are taking your driving test you learn your highway code, you take lessons, you spend a lot of time practising, so that you are likely to pass first time. You do everything you can to ensure the best possible outcome.

Even arranging to have a friend round for a meal takes quite some time in the exchange of calls or emails to fix the date, then deciding on the menu, shopping, cooking and, if you are like me, desperately tidying up so you are not embarrassed when they walk through the door, in comparison to the time you spend enjoying your friend's company.

Being born is the most important event of your baby's life, and giving birth is one of the most important events of yours.

It can either be traumatic or empowering according to the decisions you make and how you set it up. One of the most important parts of your preparation is the practice.

Each time you practise you let go a little more, and a little more, of the stresses, the tensions, the worries and the concerns. It has a cumulative effect. So many times, people have told me after their birth that if only they had realised how important it was, they would have done much more practice of the relaxations beforehand.

Do one of the relaxations in this chapter each night before you go to sleep, and just after you have done a few minutes of breathing practice. Ideally, have them read to you by your partner. The only skill needed to use these scripts extremely effectively is to be able to read slowly and gently, leaving plenty of pauses. Relaxing may sound so simple, but like anything, the more you practise the better you get at it.

As a tip for guidance about reading the scripts, leave one second between sentences and three seconds between paragraphs, and read very slowly in between. If you think you are reading slowly, read twice as slowly next time.

The first script, *Sssoften Relaxation*, starts with a relaxation of the head and face. We can hold a great deal of tension in our face: around our eyes, in our jaws, perhaps in our shoulders and neck. If we release the tension in the head and face, then the rest of the body relaxes in sympathy, so it helps us to release tension in the whole of the body. Releasing the area of the jaw particularly relates to relaxing the area of the pelvis.

Then there follows a section where we learn to use a word that can quickly trigger release of tension when we give birth.

So settle yourself comfortably in a quiet place, take a long, slow 'up' breath, and begin the first relaxation that follows (*Sssoften Relaxation,* page 70). Then open your eyes and be aware of your surroundings again. That is a lovely simple relaxation to start with.

*Stroking Relaxation* is the next script (page 72). It incorporates the sense of touch into your practice.

We live in a very un-touchy society, and yet touch, for many people, is so comforting and therapeutic. If you feel down, it comforts you if somebody puts their arm around your shoulders. Touch is important at any time, and it is especially important when you are giving birth. Gentle stroking facilitates the production of oxytocin, the main hormone that facilitates labour. This relaxation involves your partner stroking your hand and arm. Start at the fingers and stroke up your hand and forearm.

There is no special reason for stroking the arm rather than any other part of your body, except it is usually available, for example when you are waiting in triage (which can be quite a long wait) to be admitted to hospital or if you are in a birthing pool. But if it is the middle of the winter and you are snuggled under the bed covers while your partner reads this script, stroking your forehead might be a good option. In labour it can be comforting to have your abdomen stroked. Stroking is relaxing on its own, but if you practise it while you are deeply relaxed, you learn to associate the touch with a much deeper relaxation than the touch on its own would convey. So when you feel your arm being stroked while you are giving birth, it takes you into a very deep state of relaxation.

Some people may not like being stroked. If it tickles, ask your partner to stroke a little more firmly, or they can just rest their hand on your shoulder or another part of your body. If you really don't like being stroked you don't have to use this script, there are five to choose from, but it is sensible if you can to practise this one occasionally because you never know what you are going to feel like when you are giving birth. You can't predict what you are going to want when you are in labour. My colleague Nancy Keen doesn't like being stroked. She has three children and, while she was giving birth to the first two, she didn't want to be touched. During the third birth she was asking her husband to, 'Stroke me, stroke me'. This script contains five positive statements about birth. You can use all or just one or two of them. Use them in a way that works for you, or use different statements on different days for variety in your daily practice.

Next we come to another script that also involves touch: *Calming Touch Relaxation* (page 74). It starts by suggesting that your partner rests their hand on your abdomen. The reason for this is that, during labour, a midwife will put her hand on your abdomen to feel your surges and your baby. If you have practised releasing to the feel of a hand on your abdomen, that touch will have become an aid to relaxation rather than an intrusion. Sometimes you can practise with a hand on another part of your body, such as your wrist or shoulder, instead if you prefer.

The next part of the *Calming Touch Relaxation* involves your partner picking up your hand and dropping it three times. The script tells you clearly when to do this so it is very simple. Just raise her arm about 10cm and let it drop onto a soft surface, her lap, the arm of a sofa, or a bed. It is amazing to me how many people find it impossible to remain relaxed while someone else lifts a hand for them. It just shows we need practice in something as simple as relaxation. It is also almost incredible how quickly this takes you into a deep relaxation. It's good if mums read this one for their partner too so they understand how effective it is and how good it feels. Then the script goes on to introducing colour. It is said that 80 per cent of our input comes from sight, so it makes sense to introduce this sense into the practice we do. There is no right or wrong colour to use; just whatever enters your mind. It might even be more than one colour, or a different colour every day. Pink is a very calming colour.

When you reach about 37 weeks, put up something in your home, a scarf, a piece of tissue paper, a pillow case, etc., of your relaxing colour and have it in the room when you give birth, because that colour has become a visual trigger for relaxation.

These scripts are designed for you to practise together as a couple but, if that is impossible, they are also available as audios from www.kghypnobirthing.com.

It is also a good idea to enlist the sense of smell, a very basic primal sense, when you are practising by using a diffuser with essential oil of lavender in it. Lavender is known to be one of the most relaxing essential oils and you can also use the oil when you are in labour to help you feel calm. If you decide to go to hospital to have your baby you may not be allowed to use a diffuser for essential oil in case it upsets another pregnant woman, so you would have to use the oil on a tissue or a handkerchief, but it is a lovely thing to have when you are at home.

When you practise these relaxations with your partner, their voice will also become an anchor for relaxation so that, when you hear those words of encouragement, spoken softly and gently while you are in labour, that sound will automatically take you into a state of deep relaxation because of the practice you have done in pregnancy.

At the end of each relaxation you can choose to either drift off to sleep or become awake and alert again. If you are using the script before you go to sleep, just omit or say to yourself at the beginning that you will ignore the part that tells you to become alert, and sink into a deep and comfortable sleep.

## SSSOFTEN RELAXATION

Just allow your breathing to slow down and deepen; so comfortable and so serene. As I speak, allow your eyes to close, gently and easily, so that you start to release, serenely and peacefully. Breathe comfortably, slowly and deeply. Allow your body to sink … deeply soothing … completely comfortable …

There may be sounds around you, but they are all part of this wonderful experience, as you simply focus on my voice.

Now let the softness in your eyelids spread upwards to your forehead so that it too becomes smooth and comfortable. Enjoy the feeling of comfort and wellbeing.

Just pause for a short time, and now allow the softness to spread naturally from your forehead, flow down over the bridge of your nose, then in and around your eyes, and on downwards through your cheeks, to your jaw, and your neck, everything releasing as the soothing comfort gently spreads.

Now allow your mouth to release as well, so that it is entirely soft and comfortable, with your lips and your eyes gently smiling.

Feel your tongue resting completely naturally in your mouth, so that now your whole face and head feel calm and serene. Enjoy the feeling of comfort and wellbeing.

Finally, allow your shoulders to release and sink to their natural level, so that your whole body is serene, limp and at ease, and your breathing is soft and slow.

Imagine now that you are looking up at the sky. The sky is overcast with dark, heavy clouds. The clouds represent any worries you may have about birth. Now a ray of bright sunlight shines through the clouds, shining directly down on you. You can feel its warmth, and you remember that, above the clouds, all is sunshine, warmth and softness.

In a moment I am going to say the word 'sssoften'. Are you ready now? Sssoften! As you hear the gentle sound of the word sssoften, feel yourself rising gently higher and higher along the ray of sunshine, easily, lightly. Are you ready now? Sssoften! Sssoften! You hear the air rushing beside you and, as you approach the clouds, the ray of sunshine protects you – Sssoften! – and you rise through the clouds to the softness and light above the clouds. All the fears and negative ideas drop away, so soft, so warm, so safe, so comfortable; to the place of confidence, calm and comfort. Enjoy the experience of confidence, of calm and of comfort.

Now you look down through the clouds along that ray of sunshine and see yourself where you are now with the sunshine shining on you. All the confidence, calm and comfort flow into your body and mind where you are now. Notice that, as you see yourself, you feel confident, calm and comfortable. All is well. All is very well. Your subconscious mind has absorbed the confidence, calm and comfort permanently.

Now these changes have been made, float gently back into your body again as you sit where you are now. And now rest in the sure knowledge that this wonderful calm serenity is there for you when you give birth to our baby so gently and naturally, filled with confidence and trust.

You realise your body has been specially designed to give birth naturally, easily and comfortably, so you look forward to giving birth to our baby as the most wonderful and empowering experience, and meeting our baby happily and calmly.

Next time you will go even more deeply, easily and quickly into peace and serenity, knowing how good it feels and how comfortable it is, and each time you hear the word, Sssoften! you are filled with confidence, calm and comfort. Now open your eyes and take your time fully becoming aware of your surroundings, gently and calmly.

## STROKING RELAXATION

Gently and easily allow your eyes to close, so that you can focus better on my voice. Just allow your breathing to slow down and deepen ... so comfortable and so serene.

Now feel the weight of your feet on the floor (or on the bed). As you focus on your feet, feel any stress or tension flow irresistibly down out of your body through your feet, down into the ground, to be replaced by a wave of relaxation and serenity ... so you feel relief and comfort, as a feeling of warmth and wellbeing permeates your whole being. Your breath becomes slower and deeper, slower and deeper. Comfort and wellbeing.

*(Start stroking her hand and arm, speaking slowly and calmly.)*

As I speak, I'll begin to stroke your hand very gently and softly. Just allow yourself to enjoy the pleasant sensation in your hand, the soothing, relaxing touch. Your hand feels as though it is safely enveloped in a silk or velvet glove, endorphins spreading throughout your body ... So soft, so warm, so safe, so comfortable.

Now you notice that all feeling begins to fade away from your hand. You can feel my touch, but all you are aware of in your hand is warmth and comfort, maybe a slight tingling, and your hand becomes increasingly numb. It rests relaxed, loose and senseless ...

As I keep stroking, so the feeling in your hand becomes less and less. You feel so relaxed, because you know your hand is completely safe and comfortable.

Gradually your hand becomes more and more free from sensation ... until you feel nothing at all in your hand.

Now you can apply this warm, comfortable numbness wherever you wish to in your body. All you have to do is just bring to mind the part of your body that will be free from sensation, and all feeling gradually fades gently away, fades gently away. Enjoy this sensation. Comfort and wellbeing.

As you are now very relaxed, just spend a little time to:

1 Allow a feeling of wellbeing and empowerment to permeate your body, and fill you with confidence at the birth of our baby.

2 Appreciate the power of your maternal intuition, that guides and protects you and our baby through labour and birth.

3 Grow in confidence knowing that your body has been made to give birth efficiently and calmly.

4 Allow your body to loosen and relax, as you will during your labour and our baby's natural birth.

5 Allow your mind and body to grow in harmony for a swift and gentle labour and birth.

*(Pause. When enough time has passed, stop stroking.)*

This has been a very special time as you become so relaxed and happy in the knowledge of the fulfilment that is before you, in the birth of our baby. You now know you are able to affect your body as you wish. In a minute it will be time to come back to me in this room, bringing the calm confidence with you, wonderfully relaxed, refreshed and empowered, confident that our baby's birth will be relaxed and healthy, calm and quick. Knowing that, next time we do this, you will relax even more deeply, your confidence will be even more profound, and you will quickly become even more free of all sensation ... And now, in your own time, open your eyes – wide awake and alert.

## CALMING TOUCH RELAXATION

*(Gently rest your hand on your partner's abdomen.)*

As my hand rests on your abdomen, so your eyes close, and your eyelids rest just as lightly, just as gently on your cheeks, as your breathing slows and deepens … slows and deepens. There may be sounds around you but they are all part of this wonderful experience, as you simply focus on my voice.

Allow your attention to rest on your eyes, soothing and calm, on your jaw, soothing and calm, on your shoulders, soothing and calm, on your abdomen, soothing and calm, on your feet, soothing and calm, on any other part of your body wherever you choose soothing and calm. Your whole body sinks into deep and comfortable tranquillity, deeper and deeper, so comfortable, so easy; a wonderful feeling of wellbeing. Every organ and cell within you functioning healthily, easily, restfully. Calm and serenity flowing throughout your body and filling your mind with confidence and trust. And every time you feel a hand on your abdomen, you will immediately go twice as deeply into calm serenity.

Now observe that your breathing has slowed … and deepened. Breathing in … and breathing out …, breathing in … and breathing out … so comfortable, so profound.

*(Take hand from abdomen and place on wrist)*

Now I shall gently raise your arm a little. Let me take all the weight.

*(Raise arm around 10cm)*

Feel your arm gently rising as I take all the weight and raise it for you. Notice how heavy it feels. It feels very, very good just to allow me to lift your arm, knowing that, in a minute, when I gently let go and let it flop down onto your lap, your body and mind will soften and release more and more.

*(Let go of arm).*

Now again, just notice your arm rising easily as I raise it for you. *(Raise arm)*

And when I drop it you will be in a state of very deep peace and ease. *(Release arm)*

So deeply calm and comfortable. Deeper and deeper. And again, now, I'm gently raising your arm. *(Raise arm)*

As I let go, you go many times deeper. *(Let go of arm)*

Deeper and deeper. More and more serene. So comfortable. So profound.

As you rest, so comfortably and calmly, notice a colour gradually entering your mind ... A colour that carries with it all the calmness and comfort that you have just created ... A colour that you can bring to mind at any time, any time at all, to take you powerfully into this wonderful deeply comfortable state that you are experiencing now. And each time you bring this colour to mind you become more calm, more comfortable and confident, and you feel happy and positive about the birth of your baby.

Enjoy this unique comfort and serenity that you have created in your body and in your mind. Deeper and deeper. Know now that this easy, deep comfort and calm is there for you as you, your body, and your baby share the empowering experience of labour and birth, gently, confidently, calmly. You realise your body has been specially designed to give birth naturally, easily and comfortably, so you look forward to giving birth to our baby as the most wonderful and empowering experience, and meeting our baby happily and calmly.

Allow this feeling of intuitive confidence and calm to remain with you as you gradually become aware of your surroundings again and, in your own time, open your eyes, calm and aware, awake and confident, both now and when you gently and naturally give birth to our baby.

The next relaxation was requested by a KGH mother. She told me that she was so busy with work and working through her 'to do' list before the baby arrived, that she had been too busy to really enjoy her pregnancy, and wished she had taken time to appreciate this very special time. I hope it helps you enjoy your pregnancy.

## GARDEN OF PREGNANCY RELAXATION

Now imagine you are going to work. You have so much to do that you are hurrying, thinking of all the jobs that need to be accomplished in so little time. In your mind you are already at work, trying to get through as many tasks as possible, but there always seem to be more, and so little time.

Then a tiny kick within you reminds you that you are carrying a baby. A baby that is growing every day. A baby that is now part of you but will soon be its own small person. You stop for a moment and remember the miracle of pregnancy and birth. This is such a special time, such a relatively short time, a time to be relished and enjoyed. As you pause to consider this you remember that your thoughts, your emotions, and everything you do affect your baby. These thoughts, these emotions and these actions will affect how your baby is born, and how your baby is born is the most important event in the whole of its life, and one of the most important events in yours.

As you pause you look around, and find that you are in a beautiful garden. You hadn't even noticed it before because you were rushing through so fast, but now you look around and notice how very beautiful it is. You begin to wander along the enticing paths of the garden, enjoying every fascinating turn, noticing the flicker of sunlight through the trees, wandering past the sunny borders and noticing the beautiful flowers, their fabulous colours, their fragrant perfumes.

You pause again to pick a flower. Notice the colour, enjoy the perfume, and say to yourself, 'Pause, pause.'

You wander a little further and are drawn to pick another flower. Notice the colour, enjoy the perfume, and say to yourself, 'Enjoy, enjoy.'

Further on you notice another flower that particularly attracts you. You reach down and pick it, noticing the colour, enjoying the perfume, and saying to yourself, 'Grateful, grateful.'

One by one you pick a posy of beautifully coloured flowers with a fabulous perfume, and each of those flowers brings to mind different words:

'Positive, positive.'

'Happy, happy.'

'Peace, peace.'

As you wander through the garden, carrying your beautiful posy, aware of the gentle movements of the baby growing within you, you are reminded to take time during this special time of pregnancy. Time to relish the experience. Time to connect with your baby.

Life goes on but, within that framework, there are plenty of things that you can let go of. Maybe they don't really need to be done. Maybe you can ask others for help. For the most important thing is to enjoy and relish this special time.

Notice the beautiful garden of pregnancy. This is not a situation to ignore as you rush through the events of the

*Continued overleaf...*

... *Continued from page 77*

day. This is a beautiful and miraculous progression. This is a special, positive, unique time. As you wake in the morning, as you pause throughout the day, as you drift off to sleep at night, take three gentle, slow breaths, and say positive words to yourself:

Enjoy, enjoy, enjoy

Grateful, grateful, grateful

Positive, positive, positive

Empowering, empowering, empowering

Happy, happy, happy

Calm, calm, calm.

Share this experience and this relationship with your baby and with your partner, and take time to enjoy it to the full.

Remember the joy of that beautiful garden and the wonderful feeling of pausing to enjoy it as you come gradually back to the present, knowing that each time you do this your appreciation of your baby and this wonderful time of pregnancy will increase.

And now:

Begin to become aware of the room around you.

Notice the sounds around you.

Notice your eyelids beginning to flutter.

Gently open your eyes and come back to the present.

The last relaxation is designed to help you manage your own comfort levels during labour and birth, by practising techniques to dial up your level of comfort.

## YOU ARE IN CONTROL RELAXATION

Make yourself comfortable, settle down, close your eyes and take 3 deep breaths all the way in through your nose and all the way out through very slightly parted lips so you can feel the breath moving between them.

Now let your body soften, your mind become calm and peaceful, as you get the wonderful feeling of floating in your own space.

Let your body and mind together drift deeper and deeper as your body softens and your mind becomes so very calm.

Deeper and deeper. Soft and calm.

Feeling really, really at ease.

Imagine yourself at home where you feel safe and comfortable, sitting and looking at your screen, whether mobile, laptop, tablet or desktop. See yourself there with all the familiar things around you, all in their place. You are idly surfing the web looking for something interesting, when you see the words:

'Effective, do it yourself, drug-free pain control.'

This idea fascinates you; the idea that you can control pain effectively by yourself.

You click on the link, and up come pictures of different sets of controls – there is a slider with touch control, or it might be a dial with a hand that you can move round like a clock, or any other sort of control.

It's your choice. Each one has the words, 'pain control' above it. Look at the screen, and take your time to decide which one you feel most comfortable using, and then click on it.

*Continued overleaf...*

*... Continued from page 79*

The screen changes. Now there is only the control you have chosen on the screen, and it has a scale on it. It might be the numbers 10 – 0, with 10 indicating intense pain, and 0 being total comfort. It might be a progression of colours, with deep red indicating intense pain, and soft calming blue at the other end being total comfort. Whichever it is, you are in control. Watch as you move the slider or the dial to red or the colour ten, and then reverse the process and bring it down to soft blue or zero. You are in control.

Notice what happens as you work the controls. Feel your fingers touch the controls. Watch the numbers change: 10, 9, 8, 7, 6, 5, 4, 3, 2, 1, 0. Or watch the colour change: deep red, red, light red, pink, merging into blue, soft calming blue. Notice the feeling of comfort as you move the control towards 0 or soft, calming blue. You are in control.

Spend some time enjoying the feeling of comfort and control, comfort and control.

There is a very simple and effective way of anchoring that wonderful feeling of comfort and control in your mind and in your body. Just press together the thumb and whichever finger you choose of the same hand. Do it now. Feel the sensation. Remember the comfort. You are in control.

That simple touch of finger and thumb takes you straight back to the place of comfort and control. With that simple touch you are in front of your control, and moving it to the comfort position, to 0 or soft blue.

You are now in control of your mind and body with an anchor to bring you back to this experience at any time.

From now on you will be able to return at any time to this screen, the control you chose, and the accompanying soft blue or the number 0 to bring you the experience of comfort.

Remember this very clearly – your screen and your control – which you carry everywhere in your mind, always at your disposal, to be used instantly when needed. Now press your forefinger and thumb together briefly for a second or two, as you see the screen in your mind and know you can bring any pain down using your control.

Now, whenever you want to reduce pain and increase comfort, just press your finger and thumb together again, (you will call this action your Anchor in future) which will immediately bring you back to your screen, ready to take control as you have learnt.

When you go into labour, you will now be in control of the experience. Just use your Anchor and your own special control unit.

So with the wonderful knowledge that you can now use your Anchor and screen to put you in control of your experience, let your body float back into the room where you were when you started.

Take a deep breath now as with your Anchor, screen and control system deep in your memory, to use when you need it, smiling gently, open your eyes.

## Practising relaxation

You may want to use some of these relaxations in early labour, but it is most important to use them for practice beforehand, because every time you practise, you learn to release more, and let go of any stress and worry about birth.

You can use these scripts perfectly well on your own with very minor modifications. You can also practise remotely with your partner online. If you want to listen to them when your partner is not available, you can download them as audios from kghb.org/relaxation using the download code KGHAUDIO.

## *Takeaways*

* Up breathing enables the body and mind to work together efficiently and comfortably during labour.
* Down breathing works with your body as your baby moves into the world.
* The *Sssoften Relaxation* is calming and effective in helping you prepare for a positive birth.
* The *Stroking Relaxation* introduces the sense of touch to your practice.
* The *Calming Touch Relaxation* adds the sense of sight to your practice.
* The *Garden of Pregnancy Relaxation* helps you to slow down and enjoy your pregnancy. Make the most of this special time.
* The *You Are in Control Relaxation* helps you deal with pressure or coercion.
* All these relaxations have triggers for relaxation that you can use very effectively in labour because of the practice you have done in pregnancy.
* You can also enlist the sense of smell by diffusing essential oil of lavender when you practise.

# CHAPTER 5

# The Ultimate Birth Relaxation

*'The knowledge of how to give birth without interventions lies deep within each woman.'*

**Suzanne Arms**

Please download the *Ultimate Birth Relaxation* audio (see page 3) to listen to each night as you go to sleep. Use speakers so that you can both hear it, and your baby will benefit too. This audio contains three things. First there is *The Magic Carpet Relaxation*. Then there are the simple and effective Positive Affirmations about birth, which we will talk about later. You can buy a box of these KGH Positive Birth Affirmation Cards from the website kghb.org/kghcards to put up around your home. The *Ultimate Birth Relaxation* is the third thing on the audio. Finally we have put all three tracks together so you can listen to them without interruption. Listen to the audio as you drift off to sleep each night and have it playing in the background while you are in labour.

## Relaxation scripts

On the next pages are the relaxation scripts from the audio, and also some statements to empower you ready to give birth to your baby with confidence.

## THE MAGIC CARPET RELAXATION

Make yourself comfortable, and now, simply allow your eyelids to close and the muscles of your eyes to soften so that you are completely comfortable and at ease.

Now breathe in deeply and slowly at least three times and as you breathe out, say to yourself, 'Release, release, release'.

All the sounds you hear, such as voices or traffic, are part of this wonderful, soothing experience as you simply focus on my voice.

Imagine that there is a surging wave of pure serenity and calm above your head, and now imagine that that wave is going to wash down through your whole body, bringing calm and peace with it.

You feel it first moving through your head, down your forehead, releasing all the muscles; flowing over the bridge of your nose, around your eyelids and cheeks which become smooth and calm. It surges through your lips, your jaw, your mouth. Now it moves on bringing calm and softness through your neck and your shoulders.

The wave of peace and calm moves on now down both of your arms, past your elbows, down your forearms and into your hands where the wave laps finally at the very tips of your fingers like the tide on a calm shore. Release, release, release.

Now the wave of calm and softness slowly surges through your chest and down through your stomach. It flows down your back and through your pelvis as every muscle grows naturally softer. Now the wave continues down both of your legs, down your thighs bringing comfort and softness. Down past your knees and down your calves, into your feet, where just as with your hands the wave laps down at the very tips of your toes like wavelets on a sunny beach, bringing complete peace and calm.

Now release every single muscle in your whole body; soothe and release. Your mind and your body are now in complete harmony in a state of very, very deep comfort and serenity.

Now I want you to imagine a carpet, a magic carpet, just like in tales of old. This carpet is on soft grass in front of a large and beautiful tree. You know that this carpet is going to give you a wonderful and very happy experience, so you quietly walk over and sit down on it.

Now you think about the place where you would most enjoy being. It can be somewhere you have been before, somewhere you have never been to but always wanted to go, or it could be a completely new place that exists only in your own imagination. All that matters is that it is a place which is exactly where you would like to be. You are going to a place where you feel completely tranquil and serene.

Nobody at all other than you will know where you're going, because you don't have to tell anybody, so it is completely your own choice. All that matters is that you are going to a place where you will be completely happy and calm. Mentally tell your magic carpet to take you to this place, now that you have made your choice. When you do so you feel the carpet tighten underneath you; the edges curl up around you so that it is like sitting safely and securely in a cupped hand.

Now the carpet starts to rise only to the height at which you feel completely safe and happy, and it begins to move away, skimming over the earth quietly and swiftly.

*Continued overleaf...*

... *Continued from page 85*

You see ahead of you in the distance, the exact place that you so want to be. You approach it, closer and closer, until you are hovering above it. The magic carpet gently begins to descend, down, down, down, until you very softly land upon the ground in this very special place.

You stand up and walk from the carpet, and you go towards something that catches your eye. As you come closer, you see that it is a cradle, filled with beautiful and sweet-smelling rose petals. You approach even closer as you sense a small movement, and then your heart leaps as you see a tiny, newborn baby resting on the petals, and you realise this is your own baby for whom you have been waiting all these weeks.

As you bend over your baby, you smile with absolute delight at seeing it; and it looks at you with wide open eyes, and you melt with tenderness and happiness. You pick your baby up, then gently sit beside the rose-petal covered cradle. You kiss your tiny baby's face and nestle it into your breast, where it naturally curls up warmly and contentedly.

Take a few moments to enjoy this time with your baby as you pause blissfully for a while ...

The time has come to return, and so, holding your baby safely and lovingly in your arms, you settle yourself comfortably back onto your magic carpet. You are well prepared for your baby's birth as you now know how very happy being together is. Day by day your love and confidence grow, as you feel your baby growing safely inside you, and you know that your subconscious mind is gently and subtly preparing you for the important day of your baby's birth.

You tell the carpet to take you back to the soft grass beneath the tree from whence you came. The carpet once more curls its sides up and holds you gently and safely like a large cupped hand. You feel it pressing against you as it starts to lift and, ascending swiftly, you see once more the earth beneath you as you travel back to where you started.

In the distance you can see that beautiful tree and, as you see it, the carpet begins to descend and slows down, until you are hovering by the tree. The carpet comes slowly down, until very, very gently you feel the earth beneath you as the carpet unfurls and lies flat and you're on the soft grass by the tree again, but with the knowledge of the fulfilment and empowerment that lies in store for you in the birth of your baby. You are now well prepared for that day, by being with your baby already in your subconscious mind, and preparing your body to do what it is created to do, give birth gently and naturally.

You realise now what a wonderful experience you've had, how very calm, and happy you feel, and next time we do this you will become more and more tranquil and serene because you know how much you enjoy it, and understand the benefits it brings you.

Now open your eyes, and pause for a moment, and wait until you fully adjust to the here and now.

## Positive birth affirmations

These positive statements about birth are very simple and remarkably effective. You can listen to them or read them yourself, either silently or aloud. Use the different senses in your practice: visual if you are reading them for yourself; and auditory if your partner is reading them to you, if you are reading them aloud to yourself, or if you are listening to a recording of them.

You don't have to read all the statements at once; you can just read a few of them one time, and then a few more another time.

One couple had a blackboard for the shopping list in their kitchen, and sometimes the father would come down first in the morning and write one of the positive statements on the blackboard ready for when his wife came down. A few days later he would change the words as a surprise for her.

You can buy an attractive box of these positive statements from kghb.org/kghcards and put them up around your home, so you develop a positive mindset wherever you go, or carry them with you to read one from time to time during the day.

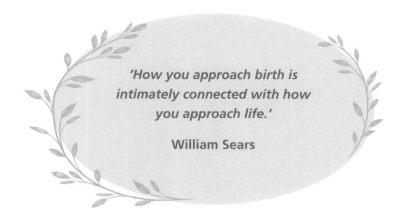

'How you approach birth is intimately connected with how you approach life.'

**William Sears**

## POSITIVE BIRTH AFFIRMATIONS

- I am happy, healthy and proud to be pregnant.
- I move gently forward through my pregnancy and labour with confidence and trust.
- I see my baby's birth as natural, healthy, swift and easy.
- I am practising so that I am confident and calm during labour.
- Birthing is a natural process of my body, my mind and my spirit, working in harmony with my baby.
- I acknowledge and trust the innate wisdom of my body and my instinct to guide me through pregnancy, labour and the birth of my baby.
- I make informed decisions about the birth of my baby with confidence and strength.
- I trust the instinctive process of birth which flows naturally through my body.
- My mind leads where my body follows.
- The changes in my body are beautiful and healthy.
- Birth is safe and empowering.
- My mind is serene, confident and calm.
- My body is protecting and nurturing my baby until it is ready to be born.
- My body is comfortable, soft and open.
- My baby passes gently and healthily into the world.
- My body is strong and healthy.
- I choose wisely. I choose to feel empowered.
- As I feel my baby moving inside me, my love and connection grow ever deeper.
- I practise profound tranquillity, and I deepen my confidence and trust.
- I only allow positive messages to enter my mind.
- I see myself holding my new baby in my arms.
- I take responsibility for the decisions I make about the birth of my baby.
- I accept suggestions that are based on evidence and logic.

- I am secure in the knowledge that I am fully prepared for a natural, easy and swift birth.
- I have confidence that a natural birth is safe for me, and safe for my baby.
- I choose the best possible caregivers during my pregnancy and the birth of my baby.
- I choose the best place for my baby to be born naturally and calmly.
- I am strong, I am healthy, I feel in control.
- I consider the evidence and make an informed choice about my place of giving birth
- I enjoy the feeling of natural peace, calm and softness that permeates my body.
- As I gently progress through labour and birth, I go deeper into peace and calmness.
- Each breath is slow, long, deep and easy.
- With each surge I breathe deeply, focus upwards, and work with my body.
- With each breath out, I breathe out tension and stress.
- With each breath in, I breathe in calmness and comfort, peace and trust.
- I feel positive, confident and optimistic.
- I look forward to my baby's birth.
- My baby is born on its birthday.
- Throughout my labour I go deeper and deeper within to my innate wisdom and intuition.
- I trust that my body and my baby are healthy and calm.
- My baby naturally moves into the best position for a natural, swift and gentle birth.
- Baby knows best.
- I feel positive and calm whatever form my birthing takes.
- Whenever a negative thought comes into my mind, I imagine a beautiful rose, its colour, its softness, its scent.
- I trust the natural process of birth working gently through my body and my baby.

- Each surge of my body reminds me that I will soon be holding my baby in my arms.
- I serenely accept my birthing as just right for me, and for my baby.
- I release more and more deeply as my labour advances and my baby moves closer and closer to birth.
- I feel calm, serene and at ease.
- I am in awe of the miracle of birth.
- Birth is powerful, and so am I.
- Everything I hear helps me become more calm and at peace.
- With each surge my breath is slow and deep, my body is soft, and my mind is calm.
- I trust my body, my instinct, and nature to lead me and my baby gently through labour and birth.
- As labour develops, my feeling of peace deepens and my body softens and opens, wider and wider.
- After my baby is born, gently, calmly and healthily, the placenta follows easily and naturally.
- My baby moves smoothly into the world, the placenta follows, and my blood vessels close naturally and healthily.
- I eat healthily and take care of my body for me and for my baby.
- My body and my baby's body are created the right size to birth naturally.
- My baby is born at the right time for a natural, swift and gentle birth.
- I have plenty of milk for my baby, and I feed my baby easily and comfortably.
- My body is designed to give birth efficiently and easily.
- I have chosen to be serene, calm and confident during labour.
- I make the best and most rational decisions about the birth of my baby.
- My baby is born healthy, alert and serene.
- I welcome my baby with love and delight.

## *COLOUR AND CALMNESS RELAXATION*

It's so easy to let your breathing be completely natural, and notice how easily and gently you are relaxing, breathing in and breathing out ... breathing in and breathing out ... deeply, slowly, comfortably.

As you relax more deeply, you notice that your eyelids feel heavier, and very naturally start closing ... slowly and easily ... slowly and easily ... until now they are completely closed.

Now give yourself permission to imagine a warm, unstoppable wave of complete relaxation, starting at the very top of your head, and beginning to wash comfortably down through your body. As it flows through every part of your body, so that part becomes completely limp and relaxed. Feel it now flowing from the top of your head down. Your forehead becomes completely smooth as it totally relaxes ... Now you feel the muscles around your eyes soften and let go. Now your cheeks relax ... now your lips ... and even inside your mouth, your tongue relaxes. Now the muscles of your jaw soften and let go ... comfortably, easily ... as you go down and further down ... enjoy the release.

The wave flows on through your neck, relaxing it and enveloping your shoulders, and now that feeling of warmth and ease washes down your arms, relaxing every point as it flows from your shoulders, through your upper arms, past your elbows, down into your lower arms, and on into your hands, the backs of your hands and your palms, all the way down to the ends of your fingers, allowing everything to become relaxed and comfortable.

Now the wave surges gently on through your chest, relaxing everything, through your stomach, gently soothing, and the muscles of your pelvic area relax, just as they will as you give birth to your baby, reflecting the soft relaxation in your jaw ... and on into your legs, down your thighs, and into your lower legs, then down into your feet, where, like the surging sea, it laps at the very tips of your toes, making both your legs completely relaxed. And now you realise that you are very, very relaxed. This feeling of wellbeing allows you to go deeper and deeper, and each time you go more quickly, more deeply, easily and gently into ultimate relaxation. Down and further down. More and more profound.

Now you become even more deeply relaxed, as you imagine yourself lying in a beautiful field in the countryside. The grass is soft and verdant and you are so comfortable, and so you let yourself gently and safely sink down and further down into the gentle, caressing grass, feeling warm, comfortable and happy. You notice, passing across your view, many beautiful butterflies, of every colour and hue, shape and size. And as you sink deeper, you become more and more profoundly relaxed, until you find yourself lying gently on the soft grass surrounded by all these beautiful colours, and completely, completely, relaxed and calm.

As you lie comfortably, calmly and relaxed on the soft green grass, breathing easily, deeply, slowly, happily and calmly, you notice that, as the different groups of butterflies come and go, twist and turn, change shape and intermingle, they create the most beautiful patterns and colours, and these colours affect your own emotions with their beauty, and your body and mind absorb their calmness and fluidity, allowing you to sink down and further down, into gentle peace.

And now you notice that, almost miraculously, the different-coloured butterflies have separated into bands of colour, so that, like light through a prism, every colour of the spectrum can be seen before you, gently pulsating to the rhythm of your body, as the butterflies themselves gently twist and turn in the air. They drift effortlessly above you like leaves in a soft breeze. How relaxing this is; so calming and so peaceful.

*Continued overleaf...*

*... Continued from page 93*

Now the butterflies float silently, separate and move away out of sight, until, like a gentle cloud, you see coming towards you the most beautiful purple swirl of gentle, dainty butterflies, ranging in colour from a soft red to a calming blue. And as the butterflies intermingle and pass around each other, you experience the energy of the colour purple, flowing softly around and through you, bringing you confidence and trust. This has a wonderful effect on your mind, filling you with relaxation, and happiness, and quietness, bringing you the peace of mind that will be with you throughout your pregnancy, and your baby's birth. So you feel calm and confident, and these wonderful feelings allow you to trust your inner wisdom, and drift down and further down, safer and safer.

See before you now the red butterflies separating and leaving as a body, off into the distance, and almost miraculously the colour surrounding and infusing you becomes the wonderful blue of the group that remains, clear and serene like the azure blueness of a summer's day, and this blue flows softly around and through the upper part of your body, bringing a lightness and beauty to your world, and with it a gentle and soft happiness. A feeling of calmness, peace and wellbeing envelopes and soothes you, down and further down.

You notice that your breathing becomes even more gentle and easy, and this wonderful blue is in complete harmony with the area of your neck, your shoulders, and your throat, as they relax more and more, and become softer and softer. You use gentle and positive words, in your inner conversations and when you speak to your baby, and you feel as though all your muscles have completely softened. You feel relaxed and weightless ... a profound feeling of wellbeing and trust.

Now a flight of yellow butterflies silently joins the blue butterflies, dancing and turning in the soft breeze, which turns the colour around you to the gentle green of spring, the time of new beginnings, just as your body is so naturally and healthily vibrant with new life; and this mingling of the yellow and blue butterflies, each vanishing as separate colours, permeates you with the energy of green, a green that gladdens and relaxes your heart itself, where you feel such joy and love now, and deepens even further your calmness and relaxation. Joy and love for your baby envelop you, and you experience a deeper connection with this new, small being. With the new, gentle green you feel so close to Nature as she caresses and enfolds you. You are wholly enveloped with that wonderful feeling of calmness and relaxation which Nature brings to all she touches – down and further down.

Notice now that the blue butterflies are drifting away, all together, and only the yellow butterflies remain, like a shimmering dance of yellow blossom, which brings peace and calm throughout the centre of your body. You feel the butterflies floating gently around you, never touching, but the faint tremor of the air as they move caresses the centre of your body, and seems to flow right through you, drawing you into a state of yet deeper relaxation and harmony, down and further down, as your breathing becomes even more effortless and gentle, your muscles loose, and your body at ease.

And then you notice that the flock is turning almost imperceptibly but smoothly into a soft orange, as a new flight of red butterflies arrives and intermingles with the yellow ones, changing the colour from yellow to orange, like the flesh of a melon, as their numbers increase. You feel

*Continued overleaf...*

... *Continued from page 95*

this colour change particularly affects your abdomen, which softens even further, and relaxes, as every element within it calms and softens, and you become even more closely connected to the baby you feel growing within you. This effect soothes and softens your body throughout the area of your abdomen, and so you become more and more relaxed ready for the birth of your baby, as your mind and body move closer and closer together in serenity and peace. Down and further down.

But now the colours of the butterflies change yet again as the yellow butterflies dance away, so that all becomes a deep, rich red, bringing great calmness and relaxation which permeates your pelvic area and the lower part of your body. You are full of confidence and trust. You are calm, and peaceful, and happy, and you feel that the future holds good things for you, so you trust in Nature, trust in your intuition, and trust in the natural process of pregnancy, labour and birth. You know that your body is designed to give birth naturally, and work with your baby during its smooth passage into the world. These wonderful feelings allow you to drift down and further down, safer and safer, encompassing your entire body, mind and spirit.

Now something wonderful happens. The red butterflies in their shimmering haze quietly flutter away from you out of sight, and you notice that you are now softly caressed by a shining cloud of purest white, as if all the colours that have passed around you have left behind their very essence, and produced their natural combination of white light, in which you now rest, so gently you can hardly feel it at all, so gently you feel the softness saturating your very being. This feeling of peacefulness, relaxation, and confident and instinctive happiness, reminds you that the happiness and joy of a natural, swift, healthy and calm birth, for you and for your baby, is just as natural as all the colours of the beautiful, gentle butterflies that have danced in the air around you and enveloped you with their gentle flight, and is equally a part of nature.

So now you know that all is well; all is very well. You know your labour and birth are a completely natural process in the way nature intended ... and you carry within you the memory of this wonderful experience of the colours and calmness.

This has been very pleasant, and there is no need for anything more in this session, so it is completely natural for you to pass from this experience to a deep and happy sleep, waking at the right time, joyful, refreshed, and relaxed, and looking forward with confidence and trust to your baby arriving so naturally, gently and calmly. If that is how you would like this session to end, then pay no attention to my counting, and just slip off to sleep now.

If you would like to come back to a state of alertness, then follow my instructions, and the energy will easily and naturally flow back into you. I will start counting now. Five ... starting to become aware of my count. Four ... slowly taking control of your muscles again. Three ... feel the energy begin to flow back into your body. Two ... noticing the sounds around you, and one ... finally your eyes gently open, and you feel happy, refreshed and very calm. Filled with confidence and trust in your body and in the natural process of birth.

## THE TRUST YOUR BODY AND YOUR BABY RELAXATION

Take three long, slow, gentle breaths. Allow your body to settle comfortably, and become aware of the weight of your body. Just quietly notice these things for a few seconds as your muscles release.

Breathe all the way in through your nose, allow the breath to come to a natural conclusion, then release the breath all the way out through your mouth as you say to yourself, 'Release, release, release'. Do that three times.

Just allow any passing thoughts to float away like small white clouds in a blue summer's sky, noticed but not dwelt on. If you hear any sound other than my voice – traffic outside, a phone ringing, voices – pay no attention at all and in fact that sound helps you to focus on my voice even more.

Now you feel comfortable and content, it is time to go much deeper so that your subconscious mind can listen to all I say and help you absorb it, remember it, and act upon it.

Imagine now that you have just strolled to the top of a small hill. Not a large or steep hill, just a friendly hill, covered in lush green grass, soft and welcoming beneath your feet. You look down to where you left your rug in the meadow below and you decide you would like to go back down.

There are clumps of your favourite beautiful wild flowers separated a little, making natural markers for you on the way down. In fact there are nine such groups of the prettiest flowers, with your blanket last of all waiting for you.

Now you walk happily to the first flowers and, as you see yourself go down, so you feel yourself drifting deeper, your body softens, any tension slips easily away, and your mind stills. You wait briefly and calmly at the flowers.

Now you go down to the second group of flowers and as you start down you feel ten times more content than you were before, so it is easy to wait beside them a little as you sink deeper into peace and wellbeing.

Time to move down to the third pretty, colourful flowers and you become many times more deeply calm than you already were, as you wait, and then move on.

As you arrive at the fourth group of flowers, your breathing deepens further, your body becomes even more still, and you are again more deeply at ease.

Wait here a while and enjoy this release.

You move on down the hill, down again to the fifth flowers, half way down to your rug, and once more you go much deeper than before, and it is so enjoyable. You have never been so calm and content.

Down you go again, treading on the soft grass and reaching the sixth flowers where you become more and more deeply at ease.

Deeper and deeper. Deeper and deeper.

Further down the hill you now come to the seventh flowers, waving very gently in the light breeze, and you sink many times deeper. Happy, content and very, very calm and peaceful.

As your breathing softens and deepens, you approach the eighth set of beautiful flowers and you go deeper and deeper again.

*Continued overleaf...*

... *Continued from page 99*

Now you walk down to the ninth and last group of flowers and as you come to them you sink many times deeper into gentle peace. Quiet, soft content.

At last you come to your rug, spread out on the soft grass, and you lie down on it under the blue sky of a sunny day and you sink ten times more deeply into calm and content.

This is truly wonderful. You have never, ever been so calm and content – many, many more times more calm and content than when you started. So you lie on the rug, calm, happy and open to positive thoughts.

All you have to do now is lie there, happy, calm and content, and listen to my voice and the wonderful positive thoughts you have. Just rest a while peacefully.

As you rest here, you realise some very important facts, and these facts give you great comfort, for they explain how right, responsible and loving of your baby you are, that you are following the path you have chosen – to let your baby decide when it is ready to leave your body and come into your arms.

Giving birth can take many forms. Just as all humans are different, and even our bodies themselves change over time, so you understand that giving birth can proceed in different ways, and this gives you great confidence.

All that matters is that in every case the way followed is the best for your baby, and you trust that baby knows best. There can be no other measure of success, and knowing this also makes you happy and content.

So you settle even more calmly as you quietly think of these things and trust that your pregnancy and birth will evolve in the way that is best for your baby and for you, with the support and protection of your partner.

As your mind accepts these facts, you are also very sure that, as well as the safe and gentle arrival of your baby, how your baby thrives after birth is also important, and this is all prepared for with these thoughts in mind. What you are doing is the very best possible and most caring thing you could. Trusting your body and your baby ensures that your baby will not only survive, but also thrive.

One of the most important things of all is not just your baby, but also you, for your baby needs you. The safety and happiness of you, the mother, who cares for, loves and is loved by your baby, now and into the future, is so important for your baby's future and happiness; and what you are doing is following a path that will be best for both of you, so that you are doing all you can for your baby.

What you plan to do is to let your baby decide when it is time to come into the world. Every human is different and every baby is different, so the right time for one baby to emerge is not necessarily the same as for another. There is no exact, predictable time. The only person who knows when it is time to join you is your baby.

The other half of that equation is you, since your body will gently and naturally release your baby when your mind is calm and you feel safe and secure. So you realise how very important it is for you to be confident and accepting about the birth, letting your baby decide the time when your mind and body are ready to release your baby, and your body is ready to soften and open.

However your baby decides to arrive, whenever your baby decides to arrive, is right, because your baby knows when it is ready, and if you are open to that decision, calm, confident and trusting, your baby will come when it decides.

*Continued overleaf...*

... *Continued from page 101*

Remember that there are only successes in childbirth – every new baby is a wonderful success – so however your baby arrives is exactly that, a wonderful success, and when your baby arrives, that will be the greatest success.

Just as there are many different ways to travel, and reach your destination in the best way, so there are also many ways to welcome your baby into the world, and your body and your baby know best. So when your baby decides to come is indeed the best time, and you have taken that into consideration for their good and your good.

You are also very happy and very calm in the last few days and weeks of pregnancy and you may be given to enjoy having your baby inside you and part of you. This is wonderful. It is in fact truly bonus time to allow you to enjoy carrying your baby and having more time to prepare for the wonderful time when your baby decides to arrive and be held in your loving arms. You are truly lucky, because not all mothers have this bonus time that your baby is giving you. So it is important to welcome it, enjoy it. Appreciate this magical period without disturbance or intrusion.

You know that your baby will know when it is time to arrive, and nobody knows better. You are the expert, so very calmly, happily and positively enjoy your bonus time as you confidently wait for your baby's birth day.

Your baby is a normal, healthy baby. You are a normal, healthy woman, so your baby's decision when to come will be the right one.

You have learnt KGHypnobirthing, learnt it well, and done all the exercises and practice, so you are in charge of your body and mind, which is so important. KGHypnobirthing prepares you so well to approach this special day calmly and positively, and it will give you exactly the same support at your coming birthing. You have rightly chosen a calm, positive entry into the world for your baby, supported and protected by your partner.

Nothing could be happier, and all your practice is for you to remain calm and confident after the birth as well, and that calmness and happiness will flow from you to your baby, who will also be calm and happy – for your baby will be a KGH baby.

You also know that unless you are presented with evidence and logic to alter your plan, you can be confident in the choices you have made, regardless of external pressure, and any external pressure or coercion simply drops away. You can thank whoever offers an intervention, but, in the absence of logic or evidence, in a friendly but firm manner decline, explaining that all is well. If you and your baby are both healthy, the only expert in time and date of arrival is your baby. Nobody else. Your baby and your body will work together, calmly peacefully and naturally, to release your baby into the world. This natural event simply happens in its own time, like any other natural bodily event.

Rest calmly now for some minutes as you quietly reflect on these things, knowing your pregnancy and birth will naturally unfold as is best for your baby, knowing your partner supports and protects you, enjoying your special bonus time, and looking forward to meeting your baby, happily, confidently and proudly.

If you wish to float into a deep and contented sleep, ignore the rest of my words.

If you want to return to the here and now, listen as I count from 5 to 1. On the count of one you will open your eyes and be alert again.

*Continued overleaf...*

*... Continued from page 103*

5 gently become aware of your body as it prepares to come back.

4 your breathing lightens and your fingers move a little, gently and slowly.

3 you notice that light is beginning to filter softly through your eyelids.

2 you prepare to return, feeling completely confident and happy, and sure that you have made the right choices for your baby, and that feeling will stay with you right up to the time when your baby joins you. And now that you fully understand and trust it, you enjoy this special gift of bonus time. Next time you will go even deeper and more quickly into this wonderful state, knowing how confident and positive you feel. Knowing that each day the effect will be more and more profound.

1 open your eyes and wait calmly as you gently return fully to the here and now.

# *Takeaways*

✳ Download and listen to your KGH audio – The Ultimate Birth Relaxation – daily.

✳ Magic Carpet Relaxation: Use the audio to take you to your favourite place to experience the joy of being with your baby.

✳ The Trust Your Body and Your Baby Relaxation: Use this beautiful long relaxation to help you trust your body, your mind and your baby.

✳ Positive Birth Statements and Affirmation Cards help you develop a positive mindset and empower you during pregnancy and birth

# CHAPTER 6

# Preparing Your Body and Your Baby For Birth

You have probably come to hypnobirthing to help you achieve a more comfortable birth, and most of the work of hypnobirthing is done in the practice before your baby's birth. This chapter covers other simple suggestions which you can use together with KGH to help you achieve the birth you want.

## Your baby's most usual position ready for birth

On the next page there is a picture of a baby in the most usual position ready for birth. I would like you to photocopy it and put it up somewhere in your home where you will see it frequently, such as on the fridge, by your bed, or perhaps opposite the toilet.

Make a point of noticing the image as you pass it because the thoughts we put in our mind affect our body, as we have seen in the previous chapter. Just notice this picture every time you pass it.

## Back-to-back babies

Most babies move into the position with head down and facing to your right in late pregnancy. During labour the baby turns to face your back simply because it fits better that way as it passes through the pelvis.

## THE MOST USUAL POSITION READY FOR BIRTH

*My baby is in the best position for a calm and natural birth.*

*My body and my baby's body work together in unison.*

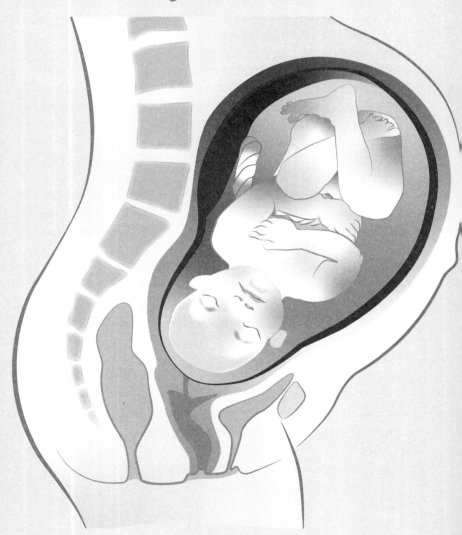

However, rather than facing the back, some babies face the front with their back against yours: a back-to-back baby. The medical term for a back-to-back baby is *occiput posterior*, or OP for short. We heard about one in Chapter 1 when we were considering the use of words. The occiput is the bone, roughly the size of your hand, at the base of the skull, and posterior means back.

The occiput is the heaviest part of the head. If you climbed a ladder and fell off, that is the part of the head that would hit the ground. By virtue of gravity, the heaviest part will always go to the lowest point. So, in our modern world, if you come home from work and flop down onto the sofa, the lowest part of your body is your back and therefore the heaviest part of the baby's head (the occiput) will be encouraged to go towards your back so the baby faces the front. If you have your car seat sloping backwards then, when you joggle as you drive, the back of the baby's head is encouraged to go towards your back. It is thought that possibly there are more back-to-back babies than there used to be as a result of our modern lifestyle, because in previous ages people would have been more upright.

Historically most people would only have had wooden chairs. If you visit a stately home, you will find that even the chairs of the wealthy people were much more upright than they are today. You can imagine people sitting on them sewing or reading, not flopping in front of the television. People would also have spent more time scrubbing floors, working in the fields, digging in the garden; all things where you lean forwards. If you wanted to go somewhere, most people would have walked, and so you would have been leaning slightly forwards joggling your baby. Babies would have been encouraged much more to have the back of their heads towards the front.

The baby's position can also depend on the shape of the mother's pelvis. For example, women of African origin have an anthropoid pelvis, and so their babies are more likely to face the front as that way they fit more conveniently into their mother's deeper pelvis. It can also depend on where the placenta is attached.

These days anything that is slightly out of the ordinary in pregnancy seems to be regarded as a disaster and you immediately get the label 'high risk'. The more realistic description of a back-to-back baby is 'unusual, but normal'. Labour may be a little longer as the baby has further to turn to get into the optimal position for being born, but we heard in Chapter 1 of a back-to-back baby that was born in 7 hours. The mother mentioned 'some discomfort' but there was no mention of pain or drugs. That's what KGHypnobirthing can do for you.

From now until your baby is born, it's a very good idea to be in a more upright position. When sitting on the sofa, instead of flopping backwards, you could sit propped up on cushions or crossed legged so that you are more upright. If you commute to work, maybe you could get off the train or bus one stop early and walk a little way, because walking will encourage your baby to be in the more usual position facing your back.

Birthing balls are wonderful things to sit on. They are just big gym balls, and the idea is that when you sit on the ball your hips should be slightly higher than your knees. You can get birthing balls in several sizes and blow them up appropriately. They can be used at your desk when you are working, or to sit at the table when you are having a meal. Because they are round you tend to move slightly, which flexes your back and helps it to stay supple and comfortable. They can also be very comfortable to sit on during labour. When you are driving have your seat in a more upright position and sit on a wedge shaped cushion.

A back-to-back baby might not stay in this position, and the website spinningbabies.com is a useful resource if your baby is back-to-back.

# Breech babies

Some babies are positioned with their head up rather than down: breech babies. Some babies can be lying horizontally across the womb or at an oblique angle – a transverse baby. If a baby is genuinely transverse when you go into labour, neither its head nor its buttocks are positioned to move into the birth canal ready for birth, and you can be grateful that a Caesarean section is available. But if your baby is transverse towards the end of pregnancy, it could be that it is in the process of turning to the head down position ready for birth.

Most babies will turn from whatever they're happily doing before to a head-down position by between about week 35 and week 37 of pregnancy. So if anybody tells you that your baby is breech at 30 weeks, this is unnecessary scaremongering. I meet many women who tell me they have a breech baby and, when I ask them how many weeks pregnant they are, they say they are at week 30. That isn't a breech baby, it's a baby that hasn't turned yet. About a third of babies are in the breech presentation at 28 weeks but only three or four in a hundred are still breech at 40 weeks. This is another occasion where the phrase 'unusual, but normal' is appropriate.

There may be perfectly good reasons why the baby has decided to be breech. We're out here, your baby is inside, and it seems very presumptuous to think that we necessarily know better. We do know that it is more usual for a baby to be born head down and facing the mother's back. But the baby may be breech due to the position of the umbilical cord, the position of the placenta, or the shape of the uterus, in which case breech could be the best position for that baby. The phrase 'baby knows best' is one we would do well to consider seriously in these circumstances as in many others. But the baby may be breech simply because it never got around to turning and space became limited as it grew so turning became harder, in which case some encouragement might help the baby to turn.

There are various ways of helping a breech baby to turn, and the one that you will be offered in hospital is an ECV – an External Cephalic Version – at about 37 weeks. An ECV is a powerful (sometimes it can be quite painful) manipulation to turn the baby from the outside, using very firm touch on your baby through your tummy. The risk of an ECV is that, as the baby is manipulated round and pressure is put on the baby to turn, it could pull the cord and therefore the placenta. If you start to bleed it means that the placenta has started to come away from the wall of the uterus so you would need a Caesarean section straight away. So an ECV is not done until week 37 when a baby is considered to be at term because the ECV carries this very slight risk. ECVs are less than 50 per cent successful and some babies turn back to head up afterwards. You may want to ask the person who is going to do the ECV what their success rate is, as there are quite big variations.

I am completely against 'trying to make the baby turn'. The word 'try' implies stress and stress is unhelpful in pregnancy because it means you are tense and producing the hormones of fear. The tighter your muscles are, the harder it is for your baby to turn.

There are other ways to encourage a breech baby to turn. You can rub the points used in acupuncture for yourself.

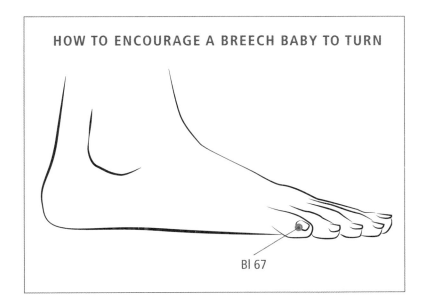

**HOW TO ENCOURAGE A BREECH BABY TO TURN**

Bl 67

Acupressure has been said to be an older art than acupuncture. The story goes that it became known in ancient China that various points on the body could be massaged to encourage and maintain health. This system became widely known, and came to the ears of the emperor, so the best practitioner was called in to treat him. But then there was a problem because ordinary people were not allowed to touch the emperor, so a system of using needles was devised instead. If the emperor was treated with needles, it obviously had to be best, so the use of needles became universal. I have absolutely no idea if there is any truth in this, or if it is just a delightful story.

You can use acupressure points to encourage your breech presenting baby to turn The main point to massage is the 67th point on the bladder meridian, Bladder 67 (Bl 67), illustrated above, the point at the outside corner of the nail bed of the little toe on both feet. If you can't reach it easily because of your bump, I'm sure your partner will help. Some women attach a grain of rice in that position as a form of massage. An acupuncturist would apply warmth, or moxibustion. For professional advice on this, make an appointment with an acupuncturist. The homoeopathic remedy frequently used is pulsatilla; a homeopath can give you informed advice on this. Reflexology can also be used, and all these therapies are said to be about 60 per cent successful in encouraging a breech baby to turn without any risks attached.

In her book *Breech Birth*, Benna Waites quotes research from Dr Mehl's study in 1994 which found that hypnotherapy had an 81 per cent success rate and was the most effective way of encouraging a breech baby to turn.

When I work with a mother and her breech baby, it never ceases to amaze me how effective hypnotherapy is. I have no idea if I am talking to the mother or to the baby, or simply relaxing the mother so that it's easy for the baby to turn. I know how important it is to say all the right things, but I leave thinking, 'It's only me talking. How can that possibly make a difference?' But 80 per cent of the time, the next morning I get a call saying, 'The baby turned,' and this can happen right up to the end of pregnancy. A good hypnotherapist can help you with this.

We spoke earlier about the power of words, so why not suggest to your baby yourself that it might like to turn? Talk to your breech baby and at the same time gently stroke your bump from the top, and down round the left-hand side to the bottom. Acknowledge that your baby might be in the correct position, because of the shape of the uterus, or the position of the cord or the placenta. But suggest that it might like to turn and that it could be more comfortable for it, that it's easy to turn and be born head down, while still acknowledging that your baby may well have got it right. So often, baby knows best. Many mums have found this to be a very effective way of encouraging a breech baby to turn.

Swimming can also be good to encourage your baby to float into a different position and if you want even more tips, the website spinningbabies.com is an excellent resource.

Remember that fewer than 4 per cent of babies are still in a breech presentation at the end of pregnancy, so it's not very likely to happen, and your baby can turn at any time – even occasionally in labour.

In 2001 the Hannah Trial considered the relative safety of a breech baby being born by Caesarean section or by an assisted delivery by an obstetrician with the mother in the lithotomy position, on her back with her legs in stirrups. Before this trial breech presentation was considered a variation of normal. When the results of this trial were announced declaring the Caesarean to be safer, obstetricians immediately switched to delivering all breech babies by Caesarean section. However, the methodology of the trial is considered to be flawed, and subsequent research has shown that it safer for a breech baby to be born vaginally with a mother in an upright position or on her hands and knees and with an experienced midwife in attendance.

All midwives are trained in the skills to assist at the birth of a breech baby but, because of the policy of delivering breech babies by Caesarean section, for many years they had little opportunity to put their skills into practice and gain experience. Fortunately, the tide is beginning to turn and hospitals are realising that breech birth had been unnecessarily medicalised, though the idea is still prevalent in society that breech babies 'have to' be born by Caesarean. Hospitals are now setting up breech teams with midwives who are confident and experienced in supporting a mother with a breech baby to give birth. At the time of writing this book, that probably applies to fewer than 50 per cent of hospitals. If you have a breech baby, enquire whether the hospital you are planning to go to has a breech team and, if it doesn't, change hospitals. It is easy to do, and you will be glad that you did.

The two books where you can find out more are *Breech Birth* by Benna Waites and the book on breech birth published by AIMS. Both these books were written some time ago and so are not up-to-date, but at the time of writing AIMS is in the process of bringing out a new version which will cover the most recent research.

# Caesarean birth

A Caesarean can be a life saver in an emergency and we are very lucky to live in a society where such help is available. However, the World Health Organization states that, if the Caesarean rate rises above 10-15 per cent it is not improving safety. In the UK the rate is now over 30 per cent and is growing every year, so over half these women and babies are being subjected to major abdominal surgery without benefit. In the USA the figure has risen above 40 per cent, and in some parts of the world it is as high as 80 per cent. We all need to be asking questions about this. If a Caesarean is proposed, check the Caesarean rate at your hospital and for your individual obstetrician.

A Caesarean is a very safe operation. It is as safe as a vaginal birth for a baby in terms of mortality and morbidity, and almost as safe for a mother. Some women have an elective Caesarean because they are under the impression it will be less painful than a vaginal birth, and some because they have had a previous traumatic birth experience. Recovery from major surgery is significant, particularly if you have a new baby to care for at the same time. The possible problems of a Caesarean birth for a baby are long term. We know that babies born by caesarean section are more likely to have breathing problems such as asthma, they are more likely to be obese later in life, and they are more likely to develop coeliac disease later on. The rapid growth in caesareans is relatively recent, so there is likely to be more research into the long-term implications in the years to come. The main disadvantage for the baby, of course, is the fact that it did not pass down the birth canal, and this is when it picks up its mother's micro-organisms which are the basis of its gut flora and immune system.

Whatever the reason you may be planning a Caesarean, I would urge you to attend a KGH course. If there is a clinical reason, such as the placenta is blocking your baby's path into the world, the course will make a positive difference to your experience of giving birth, as has been shown many times. If you are worried about giving birth, you may find that, when you are better informed and have the tools at your disposal to achieve a calm and empowering birth, you may find that you change your mind. If you don't, your choice to have a Caesarean is still available. It is the women who have a traumatic experience for their first birth and then come to KGH for their second birth who really understand what a difference it makes, because they have experienced it. They can hardly believe it will make that much difference, and then it does.

The language used about Caesareans is frightening and misleading too. We talk about planned Caesareans and emergency Caesareans. We all know someone who says they had to have an 'emergency' Caesarean. The term 'emergency' covers situations where it was a true emergency, but this is only a tiny percentage. The vast majority of these 'emergency'

Caesareans were not emergencies at all but an intervention in the course of labour where there was plenty of time to consider the options. It would be better to call them 'in labour' or 'unplanned' Caesareans. These are a Category 2 Caesareans and are probably performed after about an hour after the decision is made.

## GENTLE CAESAREAN

Recently the concept of a gentle Caesarean has evolved, where a birthing person feels more involved in the birth of their baby and finds it easier to bond afterwards. In a gentle Caesarean choices are made to try to emulate as many aspects of a vaginal birth as possible. There is a full birth plan for a gentle Caesarean at the end of this book. Some of these suggestions are beginning to be incorporated into normal practice in some hospitals, so check the situation in your hospital. Here are a few pointers about what you might want to ask for to achieve a gentle Caesarean:

- Use the up breathing before and during the Caesarean.
- Have a relaxation script read to you before you go into theatre.
- Play *The Ultimate Birth Relaxation* during the operation.
- Arrange for your doula or independent midwife to be with you as well as your partner.
- Any non-essential lighting in theatre to be dimmed to avoid a shock to your baby when it is born.
- ECG heart monitor to be placed on the side of your chest to allow the baby to be placed on your chest without obstruction after birth.
- Intravenous access to be in your non-dominant hand so you can easily hold your baby.
- Pulse oximeter to be placed on your foot instead of your hand so that your arms are free to receive your new baby.
- Conversation to be kept to a minimum in order not to inhibit the production of oxytocin and so you can focus on relaxation.

A true emergency Caesarean is classed as Category 1, someone presses the emergency buzzer, people come running, and everything possible is done to get the baby out within half an hour and hopefully sooner because the baby's heart is showing a non-reassuring trace on the monitor. The trouble is that both Category 1 and Category 2 Caesareans

- Have necessary questions asked to your partner in the first instance.
- After making the incision allow time for the baby to birth itself to replicate as far as possible a vaginal birth and to allow fluid to drain from the baby's lungs.
- The drape to be lowered and the head of the bed tilted if possible as the baby is born so you can see your baby being born if that is your choice.
- Arrange for a lotus birth* in order to facilitate optimal cord clamping and cutting so that all your baby's blood is returned to its body before the cord is clamped and cut.
- Facilitate immediate skin-to-skin contact by asking for your baby to be passed straight to you at birth.
- Ask for your baby to kept warm by being covered with blankets on your chest.
- Request respectful quietness during the whole process, as far as possible.
- Ask for your baby to remain with you, skin-to-skin at all times, for a minimum of one hour after birth for bonding and the establishment of breastfeeding. Initial checks can be done in your arms. Weighing can be done afterwards.

*A lotus birth is when the placenta is removed and placed in a bowl beside the baby without cutting the cord. This allows the surgeon to start to suture the incision as soon as possible to minimise the risk of infection without depriving the baby of a percentage of its own blood by clamping and cutting the cord early.

get the label 'emergency', which is inaccurate and frightening. You can find excellent information about Caesareans in the book *Why Caesareans Matter* by Clare Goggin.

## Positions for giving birth

This is a very important section so please read it carefully and take note.

Women worry about length of pregnancy, big babies, health of placenta and all sorts of things that we will cover later. We have already talked about the most important thing, your state of mind, but the two most important physical things are position and relaxation. You already have the tools to achieve a relaxed state of mind and body in Chapters 4 and 5. Here we will look at the other important factor – position.

In the UK, over 80 per cent of women still give birth on a bed, many of those on their backs or semi recumbent, which is the least efficient and most uncomfortable position.

When did you last lie flat on your back to do a poo? It is even more ridiculous to lie flat on your back to expel a baby, which is considerably larger, from your body.

If you were out in the country and needed to open your bowels you would retire behind a hedge and would you stand there scratching your head wondering what position to take? No. You would squat. Your body knows what to do. Equally well your body knows what to do when you are giving birth, the only difference is that you haven't done it before so your conscious mind can get in the way.

The trouble is that we only see birth on TV or in movie dramas when the woman is flat on her back, so we assume that's the right way to do it. It isn't.

Consider first whether you are working with gravity. If you are on your hands and knees your vagina is pointing downwards so you are working with the help of gravity. If you are upright your vagina is pointing downwards so you are working with the help of gravity. If you are flat on your back or semi recumbent your vagina is pointing upwards so you are working against gravity and you have to push your baby uphill. Simple, isn't it?

Now let's look at your pelvic capacity. Your pelvic capacity can vary by up to 30 per cent depending on your position. That's the difference between an 8lb and a more than 10lb baby. Please be careful testing this when you are pregnant. Sitting on a low stool or kneeling as you would in a birthing pool is just as good to demonstrate the difference. Wriggle your hips a little and you can feel how flexible they are and that the different bones can move independently. Why? Because your pelvis is designed to give birth to a baby. Look at the picture of your coccyx on page 120: the five flexible little bones at the base of your spine. Normally they curve inwards. As your baby's head passes through your pelvis they curve outwards to make more room. The trouble is that, if you are on your back or semi recumbent, the bones of the coccyx can't move so they are sticking up into the pelvic cavity and making it even smaller.

Some babies, of course, are born by assisted delivery, forceps or ventouse, and an episiotomy is often performed before an assisted delivery. The mother is put on her back with her legs in stirrups, as this makes the procedure much easier for the obstetrician, but not for mother and baby. A very few obstetricians will perform a forceps delivery with a mother on her hands and knees so they are working with her body and gravity in the most efficient position. This is rare, but it's worth asking for it if your baby needs extra help to enter the world.

So the best positions are upright or on your hands and knees. In many parts of the world a woman would squat but, since we

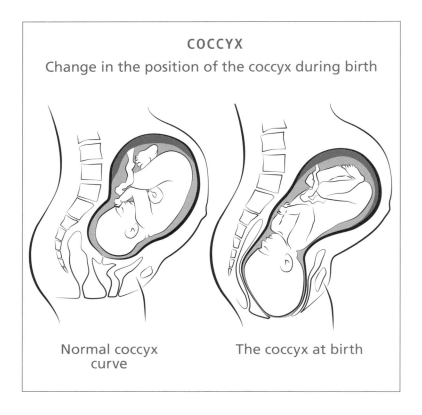

**COCCYX**

Change in the position of the coccyx during birth

Normal coccyx
curve

The coccyx at birth

are not used to squatting in our culture, kneeling with your legs apart in a birthing pool and leaning on the inflatable side is a very efficient and comfortable substitute, and you have the benefit of the comfort of the warm water too. This doesn't mean that you are not allowed to lie down and have a rest while you are in labour. Of course you are. Do whatever you feel like. But the positions I have described are the most efficient when your baby is passing through the pelvis and being born – and you are less likely to tear.

It is said that women only began to give birth lying on their backs in the time of Louis XIV, because the king expressed a wish to see a baby being born when his mistress was giving birth. At that time women in labour would often sit on stools, such as milking stools, and the midwife would receive the baby at floor level; but kings don't grovel on the floor, so it all had to be frightfully proper and his mistress lay in bed. Women of the court copied this, and midwives began to find they had more difficulty getting babies out when the mothers lay flat, so they called in the doctors more often. Then everyone started giving birth lying down, believing that if it was done in the royal household, it must be best – but nobody quite thought about what was actually best for the mother and the baby.

You would almost think a woman's body has evolved to give birth, wouldn't you?

## Takeaways

* Your baby will usually move itself into the best position for birth when the time is right.
* Back-to-back babies can be encouraged to turn round by the mother being upright and forwards as much as possible during pregnancy.
* Hypnotherapy is the most effective way of encouraging a breech baby to turn head down.
* A back-to-back baby or breech presentation is best described as unusual, but normal.
* A gentle Caesarean can make a surgical delivery more user friendly for mother and baby.
* The two most important factors for birth are your position and relaxation.
* Listen to your body.

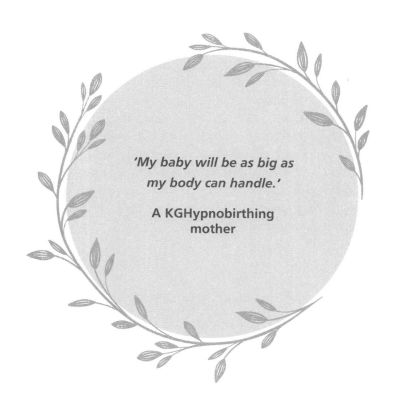

*'My baby will be as big as my body can handle.'*

**A KGHypnobirthing mother**

# CHAPTER 7

# Preventing Tearing

When I ask women what they don't want at their birth, tearing is always high on the list. Many women have this fear, and there are ways of making this less likely. Probably the most important thing to help to prevent tearing is position, which we covered in the last chapter, but using a birthing pool can help, as the warmth and water will soften the perineum, and gently breathing the baby down rather than following coached pushing (we'll cover this later) can also make a big difference. A 1998 study by P. Aikins Murphy and J. B. Feinland in New York of 1,068 women who had homebirths found that 69.6 per cent of them had intact perineums (with hypnobirthing this figure may be considerably higher). There are two more things that can also help considerably and that you can work on yourself during pregnancy: pelvic floor exercises and perineal massage.

## Pelvic floor exercises

Pelvic floor exercises are boring, and everyone nags you about them. You probably forget to do them and then go to sleep at night resolving to do them tomorrow; but then the next day exactly the same thing happens.

Pelvic floor exercises are useful for two reasons: you tense the muscles of the pelvic floor, starting at the back passage, moving forwards and right up into the vagina, hold it for a few seconds, and then release. The tensing is important because it tones muscles, and toned muscles work better. It also helps your muscles return to normal after the birth. The intentional releasing is also important because you are programming yourself to let go when you feel tension – so as you feel the pressure of your baby's head passing down the birth canal, you naturally release your muscles, and the baby's journey into the world is easier for both of you. For both reasons, pelvic floor exercises are good, so make them easy for yourself. People tend to remember the part about toning the muscles but forget the benefit of learning to release the muscles. Both parts of the exercise are important.

Programme pelvic floor exercises into your daily life and make them habitual in a way that doesn't take up your precious time. You can put a post-it note on your computer screen to remind you to do a couple of pelvic floor exercises each time you are waiting for something to boot up or download. Do them while you are waiting for someone to answer the phone, while you are waiting for the kettle to boil, at red traffic lights … Whatever works for you. Once you have worked at remembering to do them at whichever time you choose, they will become habitual.

It's absolutely true that, once you have got into the habit of doing them, it's worth continuing them after your baby is born. It gets the muscles of the pelvic floor back to normal and improves your sex life for the rest of your life. You could remind your partner that pelvic floor exercises are also good for everyone. For men they improve prostate health and erectile function. You both have a vested interest so you can remind each other to do them! There is also an app called Squeezy that reminds you to do your exercises regularly.

## Perineal massage

Massaging your perineum (the area between the vagina and the anus) and the vagina with oil softens the tissue and makes it more elastic. Many people put face cream on their faces and hand cream on their hands to soften the tissue, so we have already bought into the idea that this can make a difference, and it makes sense to prepare the vagina and pelvic floor ready for birth. Elastic, as we know, 'gives' easily and also springs back easily afterwards.

I don't think any woman likes the idea of perineal massage, but research shows that it helps to prevent tearing. I have received plenty of messages that say: 'I wish I had listened to you about perineal massage. I will next time.' So please, do it this time. You will be glad you did, even though the idea may not be attractive. If you consider perineal massage against the possibility of tearing, perineal massage wins every time.

Research into perineal massage found that expectant mothers who massage the perineum, from approximately week 35 of pregnancy, reduce the likelihood of tearing and the need for an episiotomy (cutting the perineum).

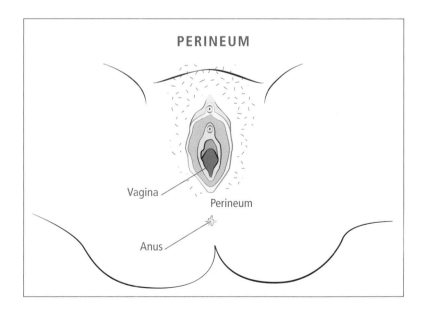

PERINEUM

Vagina

Perineum

Anus

By massaging the perineum like this once a day, you will notice the area becoming more flexible and you will become more accustomed to the stretching sensations which occur during birth.

Another advantage of doing perineal massage is that you become acquainted with an area of your body that you may never have touched before. You can feel the ridges in the

---

## HOW TO MASSAGE YOUR PERINEUM

Massaging your perineum (the area between the vagina and the anus) for 5 minutes a day from about Week 35 helps the tissue become soft and flexible and reduces the likelihood of tearing. It's a good idea to do this after a bath or shower, when the tissue is already warm and flexible. If you find it difficult to reach the area because of your bump, ask your partner to help you.

- Wash your hands thoroughly.
- Sit in a private, warm and comfortable place. Sitting on the toilet can be convenient.
- Apply a neutral oil (e.g. olive oil – NOT chilli oil), to your hands and the perineal area.
- Place both thumbs around 3cm (around half the length of your thumb) into the vagina.
- Massage the area by gently stretching the tissue with your thumbs and rubbing the tissue between your thumb (inside) and fingers (outside).
- Press downwards and to the sides with your thumbs, gently stretching.
- Once the stretching sensation is felt, hold the stretch for around one minute and begin gently massaging the lower part of the vagina by moving your thumb back and forth. While massaging, also hook your thumb onto the sides of the vagina and gently pull these tissues forward, as your baby's head will do during birth.
- Continue to gently rub as you stretch for around three to four minutes.

---

vagina that unfold during birth, and you can feel how flexible it is. Some women worry how a relatively small organ can stretch enough to allow a baby's head through. In reality it is as much an unfolding as a stretching. As the ridges of tissue unfold, the vagina becomes wider to accommodate your baby's head, and therefore shorter (rather like the neck of a polo neck sweater when it is stretched) reducing the length of your baby's passage into the world. It's not the only sexual organ that changes shape and size to accommodate its sexual function, is it? Yet again, a woman's body is designed to give birth as long as we don't get in the way and inhibit the process.

Devices have been produced to insert into the vagina and then gently inflate as an alternative to perineal massage. You can investigate these on the internet as well.

> '... whoever thought of the idea of perineal massage – we did this from 34 weeks and it gave me the opportunity to practise feeling unfamiliar and difficult sensations while staying relaxed and calm. Not easy at first but without it I think I would have found the whole labour much more difficult. '
>
> Suzie

The following exercise will prove to you that perineal massage works. You can see it demonstrated on the website at kghb.org/perineal.

Put both your hands together with the palms against each other and the thumbs separated from the fingers. Notice how far apart your thumbs are from your fingers. Now firmly massage the tissue between the thumb and index finger of one hand for a few minutes. Keep going! Then put your fingers back flat together, and you will see that the thumb on the massaged hand comes much further out than the thumb of the non-massaged hand. If it is still not entirely clear, bend both your thumbs outwards, and you will see that the thumb you massaged flexes a great deal further than the other thumb. Perineal massage works!

It does make sense; it does make a difference. If perineal massage doesn't appeal to you, weigh this up against the possibility of tearing and stitches when you have your baby, and there is really no competition. Do it! All these things add up to a more comfortable birth.

## Takeaways

✳ Pelvic floor exercises will prepare your body for releasing and relaxing when under tension and aid recovery after birth.

✳ Perineal massage helps to make the perineal tissue soft and flexible and is worth doing to prevent tearing.

# CHAPTER 8

# Nutrition

You would never dream of putting the wrong fuel in your car. It would break down. But many of us consistently put the wrong fuel in our bodies, which are such amazing self-healing machines that they continue working for years until ultimately something has to give – a large contributory factor to the chronic diseases of old age.

When you become pregnant, you suddenly become more aware of what you put in your body because it will affect your baby. If you are wise, both you and your partner will have been taking extra care for months before you became pregnant, in order that both your bodies were in the best possible state of health when your baby was conceived. As a result, you are probably feeling a great deal healthier and more energetic, so you already realise the difference good nutrition makes. Here are a few guidelines.

## Pregnancy sickness

The first time nutrition may become significant to you in pregnancy may be if you experience pregnancy sickness. Here are some suggestions.

Drinking plenty of water at room temperature with a squeeze of lemon or a teaspoon of cider vinegar can help to keep you free from pregnancy sickness and can also help prevent pre-eclampsia because, if you are suffering from severe pregnancy sickness, it is very easy to become dehydrated.

Other suggestions are to eat small and frequent meals. Have a snack last thing at night and have something on your bedside table ready to eat first thing in the morning so there is something in your stomach before you get up. Eating small amounts of what you feel like when you feel like it is a good strategy. Anything (as long as it is reasonably healthy) is better than nothing, as an empty stomach can make you feel queasy.

If eating is an unattractive proposition in early pregnancy, it's a good idea to invest in a juicer and make juices from vegetables and fruit, so that you can more easily absorb nourishment. Ginger and peppermint, taken as tea or in any other form, are both known to aid the digestion.

Other ideas are to eat something high in protein before you go to bed at night to help keep your blood sugar levels more even, and to eat a couple of crackers or a high protein snack before you get up in the morning.

If you are suffering from pregnancy sickness there is a free audio to download from kghb.org/free_audio to help you. Take a slow, deep breath and have a rest when you start to feel nauseous or try wearing the acupressure bands sold to combat travel sickness.

Supplementation with vitamin B6 (Pyridoxal-5-Phospate or P5P) capsules can work wonders. Zinc can help too, and it also has many health benefits. It doesn't seem to be widely known that vitamin B6, P-5-P (pyrodocyl-5-phosphate) can be extremely effective in helping reduce pregnancy sickness. You would need to go to a good nutrition company for this. The one I use is Metabolics (I have no personal interest!).

## Water

Our bodies are made up of between 50 and 70 per cent water so we need to maintain our intake of water for good health. Neither our brain nor our body functions at its best if we are dehydrated. Drinking alcohol depletes the water in the body, but you will not be doing that in pregnancy anyway as it is well known that alcohol is harmful to your growing baby. Making sure your body is well hydrated can help to keep blood pressure down.

## Diet

If you are already eating healthily, you can simply continue to do so and it is very likely you will feel healthy and well throughout your pregnancy.

### Do

The greatest deficiency in our diet is often vegetables. We are told we should have the famous 'five a day' of fruit and veg so we reach for the fruit bowl as we rush past. Aim for five a day of vegetables (not the high glycaemic index ones like carrots and potatoes, though these can be included in moderation) and top up with fruit occasionally. Our modern diet tends to be too acidifying, and a greater emphasis on alkalising foods can have a beneficial impact on your health. To help you, here are some alkalising and acidifying foods:

### Some alkalising foods

Almonds, apples, apricots, avocados, bananas, beans, beetroot, blackberries, broccoli, Brussels sprouts, cabbage, carrots, cauliflower, celery, chard, cherries, coconut, cucumbers, dates (dried), dried fruit, figs, goat's milk, grapefruit, grapes, green beans, green peas, lemon, lettuce, melon, millet, mushrooms, onions, oranges, parsnips, peaches, pears, pineapple, potatoes, radishes, raisins, raspberries, rhubarb, root vegetables, sauerkraut, spinach, strawberries, tangerines, tomatoes, watercress, watermelon.

## Some acidifying foods

Bacon, beef, blueberries, bran, brazil nuts, butter, cheese, chicken, cod, corn, corned beef, cow's milk, crackers, cranberries, currants, eggs, fish, haddock, herrings, lamb, lentils (dried), mackerel, mayonnaise, macaroni, oats, olives, peanut butter, peanuts, peas (dried), plums, pork, prunes, rice, rye, salmon, sardines, sausages, shellfish, spaghetti, sunflower seeds, turkey, walnuts, wheat, yoghurt.

I am not suggesting that you should suddenly become vegetarian. Indeed, meat and oily fish are thoroughly beneficial in pregnancy because your baby needs protein and essential fatty acids in order to grow and some of these foods contain zinc that is easily assimilated, but you might consider a shift of emphasis as you become more aware of your health for the sake of your baby.

Protein is important for your developing baby. The amino acids that make up protein form the building blocks of your, and your baby's body cells. There is an argument for eating meat while you are pregnant for the sake of your baby's development even if you are normally vegetarian yourself.

If you are vegetarian, quinoa, said to be almost the perfect food, is probably the best source of protein. It contains more protein than a grain, more essential fatty acids than fruit, and is rich in calcium, iron, B vitamins and vitamin E. It is low in fat, and the essential fatty acids support the development of your baby's nervous system and brain. Even if you are not vegetarian, flaked quinoa added to your breakfast cereal ensures that you have a good source of protein to start the day.

## Don't

There are many things you are told to avoid during pregnancy, but the biggest no-no is alcohol. It passes through the placenta to your baby and is known to have damaging effects, including affecting your baby's growth and the development of your baby's brain and central nervous system.

One mother I spoke to remarked that she and her husband had always been in the habit of going out for a few drinks with colleagues after work on Fridays. When she became pregnant she stopped drinking and was amazed to find how much better she now felt when she woke up on Saturday morning, and how much more she enjoyed the weekend. This was someone who hadn't felt that she drank excessively before pregnancy, so you too might find yourself enjoying not drinking.

Smoking is another no-no. Mothers who smoke tend to have smaller babies that are at greater risk of complications.

There are a number of things that effectively, in very rare circumstances, could cause upset in your digestive system and have repercussions for your baby and the official guidelines are that they should therefore be avoided during pregnancy. These guidelines change from time to time. They are:

**Known to be harmful:**
- **Alcohol,** as it can seriously affect your baby's development.
- **Caffeine,** which is found not just in coffee but in cola and other soft drinks. Too much caffeine can cause low birth weight.

**Possible risk of infection:**
- **Soft cheese** such as brie and blue cheese such as gorgonzola and Roquefort, because the mould can contain listeria.
- **Pâté,** which can contain listeria.
- **Raw and undercooked meats**, taking particular care with processed meats such as sausages.

- **Raw shellfish** can cause food poisoning.
- **Tuna** (and other large fish) contain higher levels of mercury as they are at the top of the piscatorial food chain so are best avoided at all times, but particularly in pregnancy.
- **Vitamin A** in the form of retinol from meat and fish sources. (If you take vitamin A, make sure it is in the form of beta carotene from vegetable sources.)

These guidelines seem to change quite frequently. A few years ago women were told to avoid eating nuts in pregnancy in case this caused the baby to have nut allergies. Now women are told to eat nuts to ensure that the baby does not develop nut allergies. Always ask questions about the research behind any advice you are given.

## Nutritional support

You will need a good antenatal multivitamin and mineral supplement to take during pregnancy. It is often considered wiser to take vitamins and minerals in the form of a balanced supplement rather than individually. The most commonly known multis are not necessarily the best so do your research. 'Antenatal' from Metabolics is of the highest quality and has been carefully formulated to provide mothers with optimal vitamin and mineral support in a balanced formula. Antenatal is designed to provide all the nutritional support you need as described below.

It is known that folic acid, one of the B vitamins, is important in the first three months of pregnancy to help the baby's brain and spine develop. Taking folic acid reduces the risk of neural tube defects such as spina bifida.

Most of us could do with supplementation of essential fatty acids, particularly Omega 3, and this is especially important in pregnancy. Adequate levels of Omega 3 can help prevent premature labour, but it should be taken from a vegetable source such as flax seed oil.

Our hormones turn somersaults during pregnancy, and vitamin B6 can help balance the hormones. This is why P-5-P can help prevent pregnancy sickness (see page 130).

Magnesium is an anti-stress mineral that aids the absorption of calcium, needed for strong bones and teeth. It helps us to relax, and a deficiency may contribute to post-natal depression. People are often concerned that they don't have enough calcium, but it's more likely they are lacking in magnesium, which facilitates the absorption of calcium.

It has been said that 80 per cent of the population is deficient in zinc, which is needed for growth and promotes brain and nervous system development in your baby. It is present in over 200 enzymes in the body. Zinc is a component of collagen, which is important for the connective tissue and flexibility of the body, and so can help to prevent stretch marks. A zinc deficiency can be a contributory factor in long labour or post-natal depression. Many of us would benefit from supplementation but particularly so when pregnant.

Your blood volume increases towards the end of pregnancy so your haemoglobin level may naturally go down because it becomes more dilute. This is perfectly normal. If you become tired as a result, it may be reaching the level where you are becoming anaemic, so your medical adviser may suggest an iron supplement. Vitamin C aids the absorption of iron, so drinking a glass of orange juice at the same time can help. Iron taken in liquid form is less likely to cause constipation.

Collagen helps to keep the body's connective tissue toned and flexible. Always consult a nutritionist before taking collagen supplements in pregnancy and when breastfeeding, but collagen supplementation can be an excellent way of helping your tummy get back to normal again after you have finished breastfeeding.

Some foods that can help reduce blood pressure:

- **Grapefruit** and other **citrus fruit**
- **Salmon** and **fatty fish**
- **Swiss chard**
- **Beetroot juice**
- **Pumpkin seeds**

Always consult a nutrition expert before taking any supplements in pregnancy.

## The importance of good nutrition

A mother's body will always tend to protect her baby so, although a developing baby will undoubtedly suffer from the effects of poor nutrition, the mother will suffer more, as her body will always give her baby what it needs to the best of her ability. For instance, a woman's brain may shrink in pregnancy, not because there are fewer brain cells but because the cells may become smaller if there is a lack of essential fatty acids in the diet, and the baby takes priority for those that are available.

This is just one example but, if your diet is good before and during your pregnancy, you and your baby can avoid many of the possible problems of pregnancy. Good nutrition really is important, and prevention is always better than cure.

It is important to take nutritional supplements after your baby's birth, to help you return to the nutritional status you had before you were pregnant. Many women complain of being more tired in a second pregnancy, quite possibly because they started this pregnancy at a lower nutritional status, because they had never replaced what they had lost during their first pregnancy and while breastfeeding.

Some women also complain of premenstrual stress (PMS) after their first or second pregnancies when they had never experienced it before. This too can often be rectified with appropriate nutritional support.

## Stretch marks

Not strictly nutrition, but stretch marks are something that concern many pregnant women. They are less likely to occur if you are fit, active and slim, your muscles are well toned and your diet is good. A good quality vegetable source Omega 3 supplement can aid the flexibility of your body tissue as well as the sharpness of your brain.

It is worth using a good quality stretch-mark lotion from early in pregnancy, to keep the tissue supple even before your baby's major growth spurt occurs in the second and third trimesters. Use this before any stretch marks appear in order to prevent them.

## *Takeaways*

* ❋ Pregnancy sickness can be eased by changing your eating habits or taking natural supplements.
* ❋ Use the relaxation to help relieve pregnancy sickness.
* ❋ Water is essential to make sure you remain gently hydrated during pregnancy and birth
* ❋ Take care of your diet for your baby and for yourself
* ❋ Nutritional supplements can help to prevent many deficiencies and replenish lost nutrients after the birth
* ❋ Stretch marks can be prevented or minimised by being fit, healthy, well toned and following a good diet.

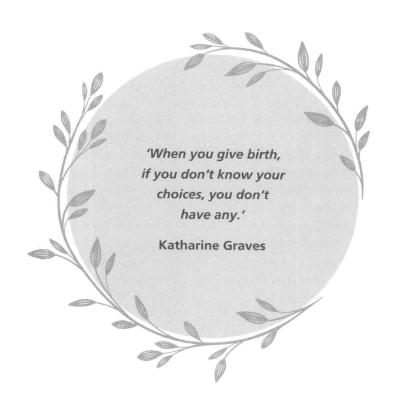

*'When you give birth,*
*if you don't know your*
*choices, you don't*
*have any.'*

**Katharine Graves**

# CHAPTER 9

# It's Your Choice

The medicalisation of the birth services in the UK and in the whole of the developed world has gone too far, and it is time the pendulum swung back. This is the view of the World Health Organization. We talk quite a lot in this book about the alternatives available to you, simply because you may not be told them otherwise. This is not to say that the alternatives are necessarily better, but simply so that you are informed. You need to know what your choices are, and the implications further down the line of the choices you make, in order to be able to discuss them sensibly with your caregivers, so that you can make the decisions that are best for you and for your baby.

You are probably reading this book because your aim is to have a natural, comfortable and drug-free birth, but you find yourself in this medicalised system, having to make choices, and all you want is the best for your baby. You may find people playing on your emotions to agree to procedures that you instinctively know are not right for you. In this book I do my best to give you all the information I can, and point you in the direction to find out more, but the question is, 'How can we change the system?' It will change because of strong, well-informed women like you. Here is an example.

## Episiotomy

In most countries in the world, an episiotomy is an absolutely standard procedure in childbirth. An episiotomy involves cutting the muscles of the perineum, the area between the vagina and the anus, to make the opening of the vagina wider as the baby is born. This used to be the situation in the UK too, but thankfully it is now no longer a standard intervention here. The first question we need to ask ourselves is, **why did women agree?**

If you ask any woman if she would like an episiotomy, the emphatic answer would be, 'No!' So why did women agree when it used to be a routine procedure in the UK as it still is in many countries in the world? Probably the main reason was that they were told it was best for their baby. A woman will agree to anything if she is told it is best for her baby. She would walk through fire for her baby, and the father would too – I know one who has. This instinct is sometimes, even now, played on by healthcare professionals to put pressure on a woman to agree to a procedure that she had previously decided to decline. Most certainly this does not apply to all healthcare professionals, but it is reported to me by women often enough that I know it is not uncommon.

In those days it was harder for women to be well-informed as they did not have access to the internet. Also seventy or more years ago the doctor was considered to be 'god'. Now a doctor's knowledge and experience is treated with great respect, but then it was almost sacrosanct. Maybe there was a tendency for women giving birth to be generally younger than they are today, and the doctor had this aura of almost sacrosanct infallibility.

Maybe the phrase, 'just a little cut' was used, and the word 'just' is still used today when a clinician wants to imply that a suggested procedure is less significant than it really is: 'Just hop up on the couch and I'll do your sweep,' etc. Women were apparently also told that a straight cut would heal better than a tear. There was no evidence to back up this assertion which was made with such authority, and subsequent research has shown that a well sutured tear is likely to hold better at a subsequent birth than a straight cut. This statement is not even logical as many women wouldn't have torn anyway so they wouldn't have needed suturing, but they all received an episiotomy so all needed suturing.

The second question to ask is, **how did it change?** Fortunately it has changed in the UK at least and an episiotomy is now only used if there is a perceived clinical reason. It changed because of two things: strong, well-informed women, and brave midwives.

Even though they may have been told an episiotomy would be better for their baby, even though they may have been told that they were acting 'outside guidelines', there were strong, well-informed women who simply said, 'No'. Their partner was not present, they were on their own, and they didn't have the ease of access to information that the internet gives us today, but they did their research and decided not to give consent to the procedure.

Then there were midwives who felt very strongly that this intervention was not in the best interest of the women in their care. It is difficult for an individual midwife to stand up to the current culture in maternity care, and midwives have less seniority than an obstetrician who may have been the person to instruct her to perform the episiotomy, but midwives would, for example, drop the episiotomy scissors, and then they weren't sterile so they couldn't be used, and, by the time they had gone out of the room and found some more episiotomy scissors, it was too late to use them as the baby had been born. Midwives today are still bending the rules for the benefit of women, and it is sad, though understandable, they sometimes do not feel that they can speak out freely.

Other midwives had the courage to put their career on the line and risk being struck off the register by simply saying, 'No'. One such midwife was the much-loved Mary Cronk, the doyen of midwifery. She died recently, but do search on the internet and read about her inspiring career. As a newly qualified midwife she refused to perform an episiotomy when an obstetrician instructed her to, then she went into the toilet and burst into tears because she thought her career was at an end for displaying such temerity.

We look back now at when episiotomies were standard and say, 'Wasn't that awful?' **What will people be looking at 70 years in the future that are standard procedures in maternity care today and will make them say: 'Wasn't that awful?'** Maybe we should be informing ourselves and having the courage to speak out now.

We can be grateful that we have a strong, autonomous midwifery profession in this country, but the autonomy of our midwives is constantly being eroded until they are being reduced to nothing more than obstetric nurses carrying out the instructions they are given.

But the real change comes from you, the women who are having babies. It is your knowledge and your courage that helps the system improve. You may think, 'What can I do? It's only me.' But I can assure you that those of us who work in this area have seen the changes that have been and are being made, step by step, by women like you.

It is our aim at KGH to give you knowledge and support to do this to the best of our ability. You are not alone, and there are many people and organisations working in the same direction as you, but I am sure it is strong, well-informed women who are the vehicle for change.

I have seen this in practice for myself. When I created the KGHypnobirthing course, I used the phrase, 'up breathing', for the breathing we do during the first, or 'up', stage of labour because it relates very simply and clearly to what is happening in the body as the muscles of the uterus draw up. I now hear this phrase used back to me, which never happened five or ten years ago, by midwives and women who have not trained in KGHypnobirthing, and it is beginning to be used in common parlance.

So, to recap, there are three questions about episiotomy in particular and a mother's choices in birth in general that we should ask ourselves:

**Why did women agree?**

**How did it change?**

**What will we look at 70 years hence that we do today and will make us say, 'Wasn't that awful?'**

Maybe we should be asking those same questions now to be sure that our care is evidence-based and stands up to logical scrutiny.

## WHO birth recommendations

In 2018 the WHO (World Health Organization) issued a guideline overview of care in childbirth. In essence the statement confirms that individualised, supportive care is key to a positive childbirth experience. The previous birth recommendations from the WHO are worth bringing to mind too because they start with the statement, 'Birth is not an illness', which is as valid today as it was when those recommendations were first produced in 1985.

This simple and obvious statement sometimes seems to be overlooked. A woman who goes to hospital to give birth is the only person who goes to hospital hoping the something won't be done. Everyone else goes to hospital to have something done, so that is the general ethos of the hospital.

The latest WHO guidelines are based on the concept that birth has become over-medicalised, and it is time for the pendulum to swing back towards normality.

Here are some of the points raised:

**All women have a right to a positive childbirth experience that includes:**

- Respect and dignity
- A companion of choice
- Clear communication by maternity staff
- Comfort measures
- Mobility in labour and birth position of choice

Women sometimes ask, 'If I do the KGH course, am I allowed drugs?' The answer is, 'Of course you are, but you are very likely to find you don't need them.'

**Every birth is unique:**

- Some labours progress quickly, others don't.

Unnecessary medical interventions should be avoided if the woman and her baby are in good condition.

**Labour progress at 1cm/hr during the active first stage may be unrealistic for some.**

Since KGH mums often give birth more quickly than those who have not done the course, this may not apply.

- This threshold shouldn't be used as a trigger for medical interventions.

The question to ask is often not, 'How can we speed up labour?', but, 'What is causing labour to slow down (or not start at all)?' Could the interventions and stress that many women are subjected to be the cause of the problems that these medicalised procedures are then introduced to relieve?

## Who is responsible for my baby's birth?

All this is food for a great deal of thought, and leads us to the important question, 'Who is responsible for my baby's birth?' And the answer is – 'me'. Mothers who come to KGH for a gentle birth, come because it works well; but it is a partnership, between you, your partner, and your healthcare professionals. Of course, you treat the knowledge and experience of your caregivers with the greatest respect, but ultimately your body and your baby are your responsibility.

In a big, busy modern hospital there will be something like 6,000 births a year or even more. A week after your baby is born, it is unlikely that anyone will remember you; but you will remember the experience for the whole of the rest of your life. The effect of how it is born will be with your baby for the whole of its life too. Therefore, it is only you who has an exclusive vested interest in the birth being as you would like it to be. People in the midwifery and obstetric professions want to support you, but they do have other pressures as well. You may be fortunate in all the circumstances of your baby's birth, but if you are clear about how you can achieve the best possible birth, and remain focused on this aim, then the mind leads where the body follows. It is amazing how often what you focus on becomes a reality.

When you are planning your baby's birth, this is the time to look at the evidence and use your rational brain. Many people make their 'decisions' about this based on social norms and the impression they have developed about what birth is like comes from the movies. Remember that the movies show drama, not real life.

These are not decisions at all, but assumptions. And the important decisions are actually the small and apparently unimportant ones made before birth or at the beginning which set the scene for how the birth evolves. Remember that birth is a natural process, and if you create the most natural environment, you are setting the stage for it to progress easily. As a mother your instincts are powerful and right. Follow your intuition about where and how you want your baby's birth to be. Your job is to focus on the birth you want.

Sometimes mothers get diverted by the 'what-ifs' and 'just in cases'. But you have a midwife to consider the what-ifs and just-in-cases: that is part of her job. If you focus on what might go wrong, that's where your mind will tend to lead you. Focus on what you want and let the midwife deal with the 'what-ifs'. She is trained in 'what-ifs'. Most of the 'what-ifs' are very rare. I am not suggesting you bury your head in the sand and pretend they don't exist. Inform yourself, consider them, make your decision, and then set them aside and focus on the positive and on where you want to be.

A woman in labour goes into herself and she is not in a place to negotiate. She enters what midwives sometimes call her 'birth trance' – an altered state of consciousness created and supported by being undisturbed, quiet and observed as little as possible. Her birth hormones flow freely and well when she instinctively feels safe in the way that other mammals do. It has been said that the best environment for a baby's conception is also the best environment for a baby's birth: privacy, low lights, soft music, stroking, plenty of time, calm. You can see a caricature of how we expect women to give birth on YouTube: Search for 'Performance: Sex Like Birth'. If a woman's partner also understands the principles of calm and natural birth and is prepared to speak for her clearly, calmly and courageously, it can make all the difference between an unhappy and an empowering experience. The person who is with you during labour is extremely important. To have the right caregiver is beyond price.

## The partner's role

Partners used not to be allowed at the birth of their baby. These days a partner is almost expected to be there. Many partners want to be at the birth, and some do not. Many mothers want to have their partner supporting them at the birth, and some would prefer to have their mother or sister or someone else there. It is important to do what's right for you. There are still some people who maintain that a father is an unhelpful influence in the birthing room, but that does not apply to KGH fathers. A well-informed KGH father or partner is a massive asset in the birthing room, and many women say, 'I couldn't have done it without him.'

If the partner is frightened, doesn't know what's going on, doesn't know what to do to help, feels rather responsible for his partner being in pain, and is producing fear hormones, they could be negatively affecting the environment, even though, as the person the mother knows and loves, she may still find it helpful to have them there. Also, they may represent the only continuity of carer she has during her pregnancy and birth, as she may see a different midwife at each antenatal visit, and a new midwife again when she gives birth, possibly with a shift change during labour.

On the other hand, a partner who has also attended the KGH course, has practised with the mother, and is producing the hormones of confidence and calm, is positively affecting the environment. Being a supportive part of the process of their baby being born can enrich and deepen the couple's relationship and also deepen the partner's bond with the baby, because they know that they have played an important part in how their baby entered the world, and birth is the most formative experience of our lives.

It's also true that people talk a lot, and quite rightly, about a mother during pregnancy and how her hormones change. But the father's hormones change, too. Dr Sarah J. Buckley, author of *Gentle Birth, Gentle Mothering*, tells us that a father's level of the hormone prolactin rises just before the birth, leading to prolactin being called 'the hormone of paternity', and fathers with a higher level of prolactin are more responsive to the cries of a newborn. One new study has suggested that men's testosterone levels drop for a few weeks after becoming a father. A mother's instinct is to nurture, and a father's instinct is to protect. These roles are not exclusive, but the instinct to protect becomes much heightened in the father during late pregnancy. The protection that mum needs is to make sure she feels safe. It is not her partner's role to tell her what to do. She knows perfectly how to give birth as long as she feels she has a safe and private environment in which to do so. The partner's role is to make sure other people don't meddle too, and she is surrounded by an impenetrable bubble of positivity.

I see this sometimes in the questions that come up in a KGH class. A mother will tell me in the break that she would really like to have her baby at home but her partner doesn't want her to. Her instinct to nurture is guiding her to a small, safe place to give birth, and home is her safe place. His instinct to protect is telling him that it's his responsibility to make sure she and the baby are safe, and he is programmed from an early age to think that giving birth in hospital is safer, although we know from research that giving birth at home is safer for a healthy woman with a normal pregnancy. It looks as if they're in disagreement, but that is not really the case. They both want the same thing: the best possible birth for their child.

I once asked a group of fathers what it was that they feared about homebirth. Was it the mess? There is surprisingly little mess, and the midwife clears it up, so that wasn't the real problem. Was it that the baby might arrive before the midwife? That was a slight concern, but it wasn't really a major problem because it seldom happens. Was the problem the birthing pool – the floor might collapse under its weight? It has been pointed out that if ten people could be in your room having a party then the floor certainly won't collapse because of a birthing pool, and two women in stiletto heels standing on one floor joist could be putting greater pressure on that joist than the diffused weight of a pool over the whole floor. It transpired in the end that the real problem was fear of the unknown. The fathers didn't quite know what to expect. It is a common fear, similar to when a child is afraid of the dark: it's not the dark they're afraid of, but the monster that might be lurking in it that they can't quite see – the unknown. Once a partner has the knowledge and the confidence that comes with it, it is often they who suggest giving birth at home because they can see the logical benefits.

If a couple appear to have a difference of opinion, it is probably due to lack of information. Do some research. Find out the facts, and you will probably find that you both come to the same conclusion. In KGH, a partner is hugely important and can make a great difference to the birth, deepening the couple's relationship and the partner's relationship with the baby.

# *Takeaways*

※ How positive change takes place in maternity care with the example of routine use of episiotomy.

※ WHO guidelines encourage individualised, supportive care as key to a positive childbirth experience rather than the over-medicalisation of birth.

※ You are responsible for your baby's birth. Make informed decisions to set up the best possible birth.

※ A knowledgeable KGH partner is a massive asset in the birthing room.

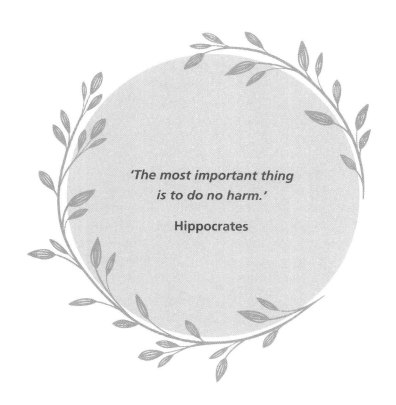

*'The most important thing is to do no harm.'*

**Hippocrates**

# CHAPTER 10

# The Team – You and Your Caregivers

Just as we discussed in the last chapter, you are responsible for your baby's birth. But, during your pregnancy and at the birth of your baby, you will interact with a team of healthcare professionals. It's important to understand the roles of those who are there to support you so that you can ask the right questions, educate yourself about the implications of the choices you may be asked to make, and understand how your caregivers can best work with you to help you have the birthing experience you want.

Before you read this section, I want to make it absolutely clear that I respect and acknowledge the many wonderful midwives and obstetricians who are providing devoted care to pregnant women within the NHS. I also know there are some midwives who have become corrupted by the system and have become cogs in a bureaucratic machine. They may have lost sight of their professional autonomy, and it is not their fault. When I go into hospitals and train midwives to be KGH teachers, the comment I very often hear is, 'You gave me back the vision that brought me into the profession originally.' That makes my heart sing.

## Midwives

Remember that it is rare for a midwife to see a truly physiological birth because of the number of interventions that are performed routinely in the NHS.

Before I started to teach hypnobirthing, I had the idea that midwives were dear, sweet things, who had a basic medical knowledge and were very supportive of mothers and babies. I want to apologise to midwives about this awful misconception here and now. In fact, midwives do a three-year degree course. Their medical knowledge is superb. They care for mothers antenatally, while they give birth, and after the baby is born. They are highly trained in natural birth and know how to facilitate it, how to bring it back on course if something is slightly out of the ordinary. They are also fully trained to deal with eventualities that may arise, and when to call in an obstetrician if extra help is needed. They are the experts in normality so, if you want a normal birth it would seem to make sense to go to the experts in normality, the midwives.

Midwives, in my experience, are almost always extremely supportive of the KGH approach to birth because their whole ethos is to support a mother giving birth, and they have seen the difference that this course makes. The reports I get from mothers are almost always that 'the midwife was wonderful'. So all the 'what-ifs' or 'just-in-cases' that may be on your mind can safely be left to a midwife after you have considered the evidence and made your choice: they are highly qualified, very knowledgeable, and have had an intensive, technical training.

Midwives are leaving the profession in droves, and the solution is not to train more midwives but to ask why. It is not because they often have to work nights. This is more than compensated for by the fact that this is the only job where you are present daily at a miracle. Midwives can feel that it is because of the bureaucracy, bullying and restrictive protocols of the NHS that prevent them from giving the autonomous woman-centred care that they are trained to do. Finally the frustrations can get too much.

One midwife said: 'I'm not a midwife being 'with women' anymore. I'm 'with' CTG machine, a set of notes, doctors directing me, and a set of policies I don't agree with.' She went on to say, 'Not a shift passes without someone saying, "How would that stand up in a court of law?"' This is a very real fear, as every midwife has known someone who has been hauled up before the NMC (Nursing and Midwifery Council), sometimes being made a scapegoat for something that happened when parents (understandably) are looking for someone to blame, and often being exonerated of all the charges against her having gone through five years of trauma before the case came to a hearing.

Is it surprising, therefore, that midwives are careful to guard their backs and make sure that they are always working within guidelines, even when their professional judgement is that it is not in the best interest of mother and baby? It is not their fault. They are part of the blame culture that we have all created, but fear is a powerful motivator. The fear that permeates our maternity services is not simply that mothers may be afraid of the horror stories they hear about birth, but fear is endemic in the NHS maternity services. The easiest way to control someone is to frighten them.

## Independent midwives

I regard this as an extremely important section of this book as our independent midwives are under threat. You might think that doesn't matter very much as the number of independent midwives is small, and engaging an independent midwife is an expensive option, not within the reach of all women.

This is completely wrong. If we lose our independent midwives, we will all suffer and the standard of maternity care will deteriorate. Choice would be restricted, and quality would be compromised.

The care that independent midwives provide stands as an example of excellence. Without them, maternity care would become a bureaucratic state monopoly, and monopolies are never a good thing as there is less incentive for efficiency, development or improvement, and no competition to keep practice in check. Our independent midwives trained in exactly the same way as our NHS midwives and are subject to exactly the same disciplinary body, the Nursing and Midwifery Council (NMC).

IMs are not wealthy women. The fee for employing an IM is high, but they provide a service that is priceless. Women say it is the best money they ever spent. You may feel that the fee is beyond your budget, and that may be true, but how much do you spend on a new car, a new kitchen, a wedding, the holiday of a lifetime? Sometimes it is a matter of priorities.

Some mothers under NHS care, may be in a situation where they have been advised to have an early induction or Caesarean section. These are the women who may turn to independent midwives for their care. The IMs have practical experience in supporting women with breech babies, twins, gestational diabetes, vaginal birth after Caesarean, older mothers and more. The safety record of independent midwives is superb.

Employing an independent midwife ensures that you have one-to-one care from a known midwife who supports physiological birth. You will be able to call them whenever you want to during your pregnancy and they will visit you more frequently if needed. Their visits will last as long as you need, all your questions will be answered, they will be on call for you when you give birth and will be with you throughout the birth of your baby, and will continue to visit you after your baby is born.

Many women have found it helpful to have just an hour's appointment with an independent midwife if they feel pressured by medical protocols and are not sure of the best choice for them at each stage in their pregnancy. It can set their mind at rest and help them feel comfortable with whatever course of action they decide to take. So it is worth calling one or two independent midwives who live near you to find out some more; they will not try to 'sell' themselves. On the website www.imuk.org.uk you can find a midwife near where you live.

## Obstetricians

Obstetricians, on the other hand, are highly qualified medical professionals who have done all the training as a doctor and then further training to become an obstetrician. When they are training they are more likely to observe and help with complicated births, the 'interesting' cases.

In the UK obstetricians do not usually care for a woman throughout her labour, unless there are unusual circumstances, but they are surgeons who may be called in if something out of the ordinary happens. There are times when protocols say that a midwife must call an obstetrician, and it is a good idea to ask your midwife which obstetrician is most supportive of normality, and ask to be referred to that one. The midwives will know all the obstetricians in the unit. Obstetricians will do Caesarean sections, forceps deliveries, and ventouse (vacuum extraction) deliveries, so they have a different view of birth from midwives and parents.

You must respect the legal framework within which an obstetrician is working. In the case of Mongomery v Lanarkshire Health Board (2015) the supreme court in the UK found against the Health Board because the mother

(Montgomery) might have made a different choice of treatment if she had been given full information, so she was not in a position to give informed consent. Subsequently the Royal College of Obstetricians and Gynaecologists' guidance for doctors on obtaining consent (RCOG 2-15b) says that:

'Before seeking a woman's consent for a test, treatment, intervention or operation, you should ensure that she is fully informed, understands the nature of the condition for which it is being proposed, its prognosis, likely consequences and the risks of receiving no treatment, as well as any reasonable or accepted alternative treatments.'

The obvious and glaring exception in this guidance is that it does NOT say you should be told the benefits of receiving no treatment. This is why the emphasis will always be on risk, risk, risk.

I remember being phoned one day by a mother who was also a doctor and who was planning to do a KGH class. She said, 'I know I have a skewed view of birth because I've only ever seen emergencies, but I'm scared.'

No doctor will have seen a homebirth, and yet it may be to her doctor that a woman goes when she is first pregnant for advice on where to give birth. This is a sad deficiency in the training of obstetricians, and also of many midwives. A doctor or an obstetrician's view will tend to be that birth is a medical emergency, because that is their reality and experience.

A midwife views birth much more as a normal, natural event where occasionally some extra help is needed. We are lucky in the UK to have midwives supporting mothers as they give birth. We are also lucky to have good obstetricians available when they are needed. Both are autonomous professionals who have their own role to play. A midwife is not an obstetric nurse who is an assistant to the obstetrician; she is a medical professional in her own right.

*'I didn't have the 'perfect KGH birth' but I did have a complete understanding of my body, my labour and the power of birth. I knew my rights and what I wanted and what was important to us as a family.*

*I felt in control and unafraid and I 100 per cent understand the reasons for my assisted delivery. I am positive and proud that I managed to have such an empowering labour and birth.*

*Thank you KGH.'*

Claire

Be sure that your healthcare professionals will be unwaveringly supportive of how you want your birth to be. If you are giving birth in a hospital or midwife-led unit, it may be possible to ask for a different midwife if the chemistry is just not right between you, but this is extremely unusual. If a stressful situation arises during the antenatal stage, an appointment with the senior midwife to talk it through can be helpful. Be prepared to change to another caregiver or even another hospital if necessary to make sure you get the support you need.

Everyone who trains as a midwife or obstetrician does so with the purpose of supporting women and babies in pregnancy and birth.

## Doulas

Some women will employ a doula to be with them during the birth of their baby. The word 'doula' comes from the Greek word meaning female slave. A doula is not medically qualified but she is trained to support the mother, giving her confidence, be her advocate, perhaps give the partner time to rest, and generally she will have a greater knowledge of the birth process, hospital procedures, what will make the mother comfortable, and the implications of a mother's choices. It is a role that midwives would love to perform but they are often too busy to be able to just be with the mothers in their care. KGH teachers are well equipped to be supportive themselves, but some couples feel that having a doula gives them extra reassurance.

## You – the birth professional

Taking responsibility for your baby's birth includes everything that makes up your internal and external environment in body, mind and spirit. Make sure you have only positive and helpful people around you.

Being a parent is a position of great importance and responsibility. You are entitled to be treated with the greatest respect in this role. The choices that you make now will have an effect on the development and serenity of your baby. Choose logically. Choose wisely.

*Takeaways*

* Midwives have extensive knowledge and broad experience. They are autonomous medical professionals, not just obstetric nurses.

* Independent Midwives can offer experience of unusual circumstances and give woman-centred care that hospital midwives are not always able to offer. The service they provide is priceless.

* Obstetricians are the medical professionals you want in an unusual circumstance, but are more likely to choose an intervention.

* Doulas are not medically trained, but are experienced in childbirth, and can be a great support in labour.

* You are the true birth professional because you are the person giving birth. Trust yourself.

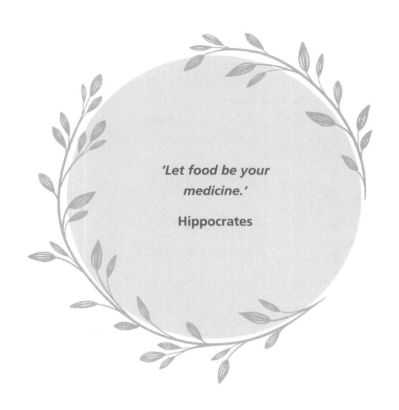

'Let food be your
medicine.'

Hippocrates

# CHAPTER 11

# If Only …

These are the two words on the lips of couples who come to me after a traumatic first birth. 'If only I had known …' 'If only someone had told me …'

This is incredibly sad and also unnecessary. The purpose of the KGH course is that we pre-empt the 'if only's' by giving you all the knowledge you need to make informed choices about the birth of your baby so you have the best possible birth experience. When you are pregnant it is almost impossible to avoid horror stories about birth. The KGH mums are the ones who report a positive birth experience, even if additional help is needed, and you can read their birth reports (and the birth reports from their partners) on the website kghb.org/birthreports.

It is the second time mums that I teach who *really* understand how effective the KGH course is as they have experienced the difference it makes. They can hardly believe that coming to a 12-hour course and practising for only 15 minutes a day can make that much difference to their experience, but it does, and it is wonderful to see.

The information we give is logical and evidence-based, but I understand it can be very difficult to stick to the choices that you have made in advance when you may be subjected to pressure, coercion and scaremongering to change your mind in the last few weeks of your pregnancy. The next chapter will help you deal with this situation.

When a mum comes to me who has had a previous traumatic birth, my experience is that taking the KGH course has always laid that trauma to rest so that she has an empowering and positive experience this time. KGH teachers I have trained sometimes call me and say, 'I'm teaching this mum who ................. What else can I do for her?' My answer is always the same, just teach her the course as it stands, and if she still needs something more at the end of it, come back to me and we will sort it out. No teacher has ever come back to me saying that something else is needed.

Mostly I teach KGH to first time mums and so for them the question of birth trauma doesn't arise.

I have heard that women who have done some form of hypnobirthing and then don't achieve the 'perfect' birth for their baby (whatever that is) can feel guilty after the baby is born. This is awful, and we work very hard in the KGH course to make sure this does not apply to any of the mums we teach.

You might think that women experiencing some form of intervention which they had not anticipated might suffer from post-traumatic stress. Research has found that this is unlikely to be the case with KGH mums. Many women have reported to us that, if an intervention was suggested during birth, lots of people came into the room, but, 'I felt quite calm.' And this calmness in the mother affects her hormones and is passed to the baby. Many mums of KGH babies report how calm their baby is, and this stays with them as they grow up. It can apply to babies whose birth has taken an unexpected turn.

The most important factor seems to be the level of support expected from your caregivers and the level of care actually experienced. This is why it is very important to stand back from the situation if you feel under pressure and know who to turn to, often outside the NHS, when you find this happening to you.

I cannot stress enough how important it is to inform yourself well in advance, which you are doing by reading this book, and even more so if you do the full 12-hour KGH antenatal course. Then make your choices and do not change them unless there is a clinical change in your situation. Fear is a very bad principle from which to make a choice, and you may well regret it afterwards.

Women who have what appears to be a normal birth can suffer birth trauma if they feel out of control, not listened to, and suffer loss of dignity, but mostly if they experience a dismissive or unsupportive attitude from their caregivers. Considerate care is of supreme importance.

The question of informed consent is very important. Not just consent, but informed consent. If a healthcare professional or therapist so much as lays a finger on a woman without consent, legally they are committing battery. Women report receiving vaginal examinations without giving permission or a full explanation. I have often heard of women being told the risks of declining an induction of labour, but never the benefits. The language that is sometimes used can be coercive too, implying that her baby is at risk if she doesn't agree.

As you read this book earlier in your pregnancy, you are probably thinking that your caregivers are lovely people who are not at all like this. They are undoubtedly lovely and caring people, but from 40 weeks onwards the pressure will mount, and you may find yourself making choices that you regret afterwards. Many women have reported, 'I didn't realise the pressure would feel like this.' I am most certainly not suggesting you ignore the knowledge and experience of your caregivers, but make sure it is logical and evidence based.

As I said in the previous chapter, the RCOG instruction to doctors is:

'Before seeking a woman's consent for a test, treatment, intervention or operation, you should ensure that she is fully informed, understands the nature of the condition for which it is being proposed, its prognosis, likely consequences and the risks of receiving no treatment, as well as any reasonable or accepted alternative treatments.' It is interesting to note that this instruction does not include telling the women the benefits of receiving no treatment, only the risks.

What can you do about this? If you have had a previous birth trauma, use the relaxation Confident and Positive, which you find on page 220, earlier than it appears in the course, and more frequently too.

We also offer you this next relaxation, which has been written specially to lay to rest the trauma of the past so you can enjoy your pregnancy, and the birth of this baby can be a positive experience.

## THE 5CS RELAXATION

Settle yourself comfortably and take three long, slow breaths and, on the out-breath, say to yourself **release … confident … positive …**

Now become aware of your body and, with each breath, you become more at ease, more comfortable. Allow any stress, any tension, to simply drop away. Enjoy this wonderful feeling of release and calm.

Just continue those gentle calm breaths and listen as I count:

**5** Allow your eyes to close and your eyelids to rest lightly on your cheeks.

**4** Rest your attention on the sound of my voice. Other sounds around you simply don't matter.

**3** Any stresses and tension drop away.

**2** Your mind clears and opens.

**1** Comfort and wellbeing. Comfort and wellbeing.

Imagine you are walking along a path in the country, alone and lonely. It's a grey, damp day, and your shoulders are bent with care and the negative thoughts that fill your mind as you plod slowly along, dragging one foot in front of the other. You shiver in the chill air. Slow and heavy. Slow and heavy. Most of all the experience of your previous birth is weighing down on you. Feeling alone, not listened to, frightened, in pain. Feeling pressurised, not knowing what to do for the best. Not being given the full information you needed. 'If only I had known what I know now, I would have made a different choice.' 'If only someone had told me.' 'If only I had realised that I had a choice at all.' 'Why didn't I inform myself better?' 'Was that intervention really necessary?' 'Why did they say that to me?' 'Why did they do that to me?' And worst of all, 'Did I do the best for my baby?' 'If only ...' 'If only ...'

As you walk along you see a door in front of you. Notice its texture. Notice its colour. As you turn the handle and open it, feel the weight of the door. Does the handle turn easily as you swing the door open? Now you find yourself in a room. The room is rather gloomy and cold, but it looks interesting so you go in. There is a hearth, but no fire is burning. The interesting thing is that there are heaps of papers cluttering up the room, and each heap has your name on it. There is also a large, comfortable chair, so you sit down and begin to sort through the heaps of papers, one by one.

The first heap says: Left Alone

As you sort through the papers you see that each one

*Continued overleaf...*

... *Continued from page 165*

reminds you of an occasion during the birth of your baby when you felt left alone, abandoned. Every single instance when this happened comes to mind as you read through the papers. Spend a little time allowing your subconscious mind to present these events to you. Breathe slowly and deeply, slowly and deeply.

When you have finished reading all the papers in this heap, you get up and place them in the hearth and set light to them. The flames lighten the room a little and bring some cheer and warmth.

Then you go to the next heap that says: Not Listened To.

All those times when you didn't feel heard or acknowledged come to mind. Every single one is written on the papers in this pile. It takes a while to allow them all to surface but eventually it is done. Allow some time for the process to complete.

Then get up from your chair and go to the hearth again. You throw the papers on the fire, one by one and watch them burn, and this time you add a few twigs from the basket by the hearth, so the fire burns more brightly. Breathe slowly and deeply, slowly and deeply.

You pick up the next heap of papers with more enthusiasm as you are beginning to feel the weight lifting from your shoulders as you continue your work.

This one says: Feeling pressurised and coerced.

As you sit down again to examine these papers and reflect on them, your subconscious mind presents to you all the occasions that this happened. All the times people imposed their ideas on you instead of supporting you in your choices. Allow time for this to evolve.

Then throw these papers on the fire too. Feel the relief as you watch them burn, and then add some logs to the fire from the well-stocked log basket. Breathe slowly and deeply, slowly and deeply.

As you sit down again you notice that the room has become lighter as the clouds outside are beginning to lift, and you can feel the warmth from the burning logs.

Now you approach your task with greater enthusiasm because you are beginning to feel the benefits of the work you are doing. You work through the heaps of papers, one by one. Each one has a label that is appropriate to your experience. Each one includes all the events that happened to you. Each one brings to mind the emotions you experienced.

As you complete your work on each pile of papers you get up and sling the papers listing those old events and emotions onto the fire. Each time you feel lighter and more at ease. Each time your shoulders straighten and your confidence grows. Breathe slowly and deeply, slowly and deeply.

The fire is burning brightly now and the room feels warm and cosy. Outside the sun is beginning to shine through the clouds.

Almost all the heaps of paper are dealt with now. You are doing so well, and the task you originally faced with trepidation, you now complete with relief and enthusiasm. As you burn these last few heaps of papers, the sun breaks through and shines through the windows of the room. The room feels cosy and warm, and the fire burns brightly in the hearth.

There is only one heap of papers left now. The one that says on it: 'Did I do the best for my baby?' Suddenly a cloud

*Continued overleaf...*

... *Continued from page 167*

passes over the sun and the room feels cold again. This heap of papers was lurking behind all the others and now the others have been dealt with you can no longer avoid it.

As you pick up this pile of papers, it feels very heavy. You carry it back to your chair with a feeling of dread. Each one of those papers contains a feeling of guilt and remorse. Each memory that your subconscious presents to you is painful. You summon up all your courage and deal with every single paper in the heap, every single idea in your mind, carefully examining them one by one.

And then your work is complete. Everything is dealt with. The relief is unbelievable as you fling those papers onto the fire, and the sun comes out again and shines brightly into the room. Breathe slowly and deeply, slowly and deeply.

You return to your comfortable chair and look around the room. With all the papers removed that were cluttering it up, you see that it is a beautiful room, and there are positive words of encouragement stencilled around the walls: **choice, consent, communication, control, confidence, calm, comfort**.

Now you notice a cupboard that you hadn't seen before. You go to it and open the door and inside is a beautiful, warm set of clothes with your name on. You discard your old worn clothes and put on these beautiful new clothes which are just right for you and fit you perfectly. They feel so good. They look so good.

You're enjoying being in this room so much that you return to your comfortable chair again and allow your eyes to close. The image of your beautiful baby comes to mind to complete your happiness and content. You know with surety that you have always done your best for your baby, the baby that you love so much, and will continue to do so throughout your journey of motherhood.

You will always do your best in just the same way for any future baby you may have. You have total confidence that this is absolutely sure. This is etched deep into your soul. Spend a few minutes enjoying this knowledge and this experience to the full.

It's time to return now, so you open the door of the room and step lightly outside. All the worries and negative thoughts about your previous birth experience have been left behind. All burnt and completely gone. The path you came on has changed. The sun is shining brightly, you can feel its warmth on your back, and you are joined by people who will support you on your journey, your journey to a wonderful and empowering pregnancy and birth.

You have changed too. You feel confident and powerful. You understand that, with body and mind working together in the way that nature intended, and the support and protection of your partner, the birth of your new baby can be a positive and happy experience.

The words that you read in the room resonate in your mind and are absorbed deeply into your subconscious: **choice, consent, communication, control, confidence, calm, comfort**. If any of those old hurtful thoughts come to mind you know that all you have to do is say any of those words to yourself. Then you will return to the experience you had in that beautiful room with the sun shining in and the fire burning brightly in the hearth, and will feel again the comfort and strength that you felt as you sat in that comfortable chair and

*Continued overleaf...*

*... Continued from page 169*

read the words:

**choice, consent, communication, control, confidence, calm, comfort.**

Every time you listen to this script or read it to yourself, the effect will grow more and more powerful:

**choice, consent, communication, control, confidence, calm, comfort.**

And now, in your own time, allow your eyes to open as you gently return to the present, feeling the relief that all those old negative thoughts have gone and approaching the future with confidence and happiness and with the words resonating in your ears and in your mind:

**choice, consent, communication, control, confidence, calm, comfort.**

# *Takeaways*

* Educate yourself so that you can make the right choices for you and for your baby.
* Stick to your choices unless there is a clinical change.
* KGH babies are often calm babies.
* Make sure your caregivers give you the balanced facts you need in order to give informed consent.
* Relieve a past birth trauma with a relaxation script to help you to leave your 'if only's' behind you.

# CHAPTER 12

# Achieving the Birth You Want

When I started to teach KGH, I began to hear many wonderful stories from mothers whose babies were born calmly and naturally, but sometimes I was told about births that were not what a mother had hoped for.

Whenever this happened, I considered very carefully whether I might be able to learn something from the experience that would enable me to help other mothers in future. I came to realise that very often in these births there had been some form of medical intervention.

Couples need information on all the alternative procedures, methods and interventions available to them in order to make a fully informed decision. The law in the UK says that no intervention may be done without informed consent. So often, however, the only information given is about why the routine procedures should be agreed to, and the consent can sometimes be assumed.

Phrases such as, 'We won't let you …', 'We don't allow you to …' and occasionally, coercively, 'Don't you want to do the best for your baby?' are used.

I am well aware that modern medicine saves lives and that healthcare providers are committed and caring people who will often extend a consultation into their own time in order to put a woman's mind at ease. The problem is that some interventions are done routinely, when – in fact – a mother might do better to remember that, very often, baby knows best.

If you find yourself agreeing to an intervention out of fear, think again. Make your choices based on facts and evidence. Remember the acronym **F.F.F**

**F**ind

**F**acts

**F**irst

You are focused on a calm and natural KGH birth, so it is very much in your best interests to carefully consider aspects of the birth you want in advance.

## The fallacy of the due date

Let's talk now about due dates. This is important. Due dates are a snare and a delusion. They are not just a fallacy, they are actually harmful. They can be the cause of extreme stress. In the early 1800s a German obstetrician, Franz Naegele, declared that a pregnancy should last for ten moons (ten months of four weeks). However, researchers in 1990 found that, for healthy Eurasian women, an average pregnancy is ten days longer than this. So the due date you and your caregivers are so focussed on is not even an average.

Nothing in the human condition is standard. We all grow to different heights, live different length lives, we have different faces, different coloured hair; it would be strange indeed if all pregnancies were the same length.

Even if you look at the apples on an apple tree, they take over a month to ripen, and if you want one to ripen early and pick the ripest and put it on a sunny windowsill in the kitchen, guess what? The ones on the tree ripen first. You would be very surprised if all the apples on a tree ripened on the same day. If you pick a blackberry that is not quite ripe, you have to pull it off the twig. When it is ripe, it comes off easily in your fingers.

The more I see of birth, the more I am in absolute awe of this miraculous process. You disturb it at your peril. Of course, there are circumstances when we are extremely grateful for medical intervention. In particular clinical circumstances, intervention saves lives. But there seems to be a tremendous amount of it these days, and we should regard it with great caution. Even the World Health Organization issued a statement recently saying that the medicalisation of birth has gone too far and, rather than increasing safety, is actually increasing the risks for mother and baby.

In the UK, a full-term pregnancy is generally considered to be 40 weeks. In most of continental Europe, it is considered to be 41 weeks. In Kenya, it is up to 43 weeks. The World Health Organization says anything between 37 and 42 weeks for an average pregnancy, which is more than a month's range.

Some babies are born at a normal size and perfectly naturally at 44 weeks or even a few days more. Some babies born at 36 weeks are completely ready for the world. The length of pregnancy will vary because the length of pregnancy is taken from the first day of the woman's last menstrual period. A woman may have an irregular menstrual cycle, and women can conceive at different times within the cycle. There are so many factors to take into account. Scans, too, are known to be inaccurate.

The date offered by an ultrasound scan in the first trimester of pregnancy tells us how long the baby has been growing for, plus or minus five days. Women may choose to have another scan at 20 weeks, which is accurate to plus or minus ten days. It is worth noting that the date you have been given from your scan is often earlier than the date you worked out for yourself from the first day of your last period. This means that, in some cases, a woman is being put under pressure to agree to an induced labour even before, according to her own calculation, she has reached her 'due date'. A woman in the UK might be facing an induction when in France the baby would not yet even be considered due.

There is no such thing as a 'late baby', but simply that women have different lengths of pregnancy. And it would be very strange if it were otherwise. It seems very hard on a baby to be labelled 'late' before it has even arrived.

Our language at this time causes even more stress. At 39 weeks and 6 days, a woman is happily pregnant. At 40 weeks and 1 day (2 days later) the language changes. 'My baby is late.' Late for what? 'I'm overdue.'

Did you know that the average length of pregnancy is thought to be about 41.5 weeks? We use the terms 38+6, 39+2, 40+5, 40+8, 40+10, 40+15 as if the clock stopped ticking at 40 weeks. It would be so much more accurate and positive to say 40+5, 41+3, 42+1, etc. Please use these terms to yourself and point out how harmful the language is if you hear anyone else speaking in this way. It focuses the attention yet again on the inaccurate and harmful 'due date'.

Please don't ask someone when their baby is due. Ask instead how many weeks pregnant they are, and, if someone asks you this same question, then reply, 'I'm x weeks pregnant'. If they say, 'Oh, so your baby is due on xxx date,' the more accurate answer is, 'No, it's more likely to arrive on xxx date plus 2 weeks (whatever that date is).'

There is only one person who knows the 'due date', and that is your baby, and they're keeping it a secret. It's worth remembering that all babies are born on their birthdays!

You may think I'm going on about due dates and, yes, I am. Our obsession with due dates causes nothing but harm, and we need to shift our focus. When you get to 40+ weeks you will understand, so I would like you to do something about it now before that time arrives.

## Bonus Time

In KGH we call the part of your pregnancy after 40 weeks Bonus Time. It is the only time in your life when you have this gift of time with nothing planned. You can read that book on your bedside table that you have wanted to read for years. You can have a lie-in. You can go out to a movie or a meal in a restaurant with your partner. All things that you will not be able to do without a great deal of expense and organisation for many years to come. (Do I see second time couples nodding vehemently at this point?) Make the most of it.

If you already have children, it's time to spend with them before the new addition to the family arrives.

Arrange a schedule for yourself with something nice to do every day, a little treat, from week 40 to week 43: meet a friend for coffee, a reflexology appointment (not to 'try to make the baby come' but simply because it feels so good and helps you chill), have lunch with your mum (as long as she promises not to mention the 'due date'), an appointment at the hairdresser, arrange to go to a movie with your partner, book a massage, organise your favourite takeaway and stream a movie. Book this NOW. This will counteract the stress that is being heaped on you from all sides, and you will be disappointed if you haven't been able to complete your pampering schedule because your baby arrives. Remember that 85 per cent of pregnancies are longer than 40 weeks, so this will apply to almost everyone.

Everyone else will be heaping pressure and stress on you at this time. My aim is to relieve stress and help you enjoy these last precious days of pregnancy. Babies of longer gestation are more mature when they are born and are better equipped to deal with life outside the womb.

## Stress

Reading this book now, it may be difficult to imagine how stressed you will feel if your arbitrary 'due date' arrives but your baby hasn't, but I can assure you the stress will begin to build. You will find that it comes from three directions.

You put stress on yourself, because you have mentally set great store on that date. This is why I would suggest that, if your baby is due, say, on 1 May, every time that date comes into your mind you say to yourself, 'My baby is likely to arrive in mid May'. This is often more accurate and far less stressful. Some midwives have suggested that it's best not to have a due date at all.

You will have stress from your family and friends. When that date comes you will get 20 phone calls from all your friends and relations to whom you have told 'the date'. 'Baby hasn't come yet?' 'No.' 'You're still there?' 'Yes' – of course you are or you wouldn't be answering the phone. 'You must be fed up' – 'I wasn't until 20 people suggested it to me.' Many mothers have unplugged their landline and turned their mobile to silent to stem the mounting tide of phone calls. To protect yourself from these well-meaning but stress-provoking enquiries, you can tell your friends a date two weeks beyond the one you were given. If you have already told them, you can easily change it by saying you have had another scan that put 'the date' two weeks later. After all, the first date they believed came from a scan, so why not this new one too? I can promise you that you will be glad if you do this; many women have told me they wish they had.

Here is some advice from a father:

*'Based on our experience, patience is paramount. Different strategies may be used to avoid unnecessary pressure. The best one I can think of is keeping the due date a secret.*

*When asked, give the end of the 42nd week as the due date. Everyone – family and friends – wants to have a date and no matter how many times you tell them not to keep asking about whether the baby has arrived or not, chances are at least one of them will not get the message and that will be enough. Being vague is pointless and will not satisfy everyone. It's much easier to publicise the 'wrong' date.'*

Third and last, you will be put under stress from your healthcare professionals. First of all, I want to acknowledge again the wonderful midwives and obstetricians who go out of their way to make sure that the women in their care receive full information before they make a choice. It is the women who do not receive this information that I hear about, because they come back to me with their questions. What often happens at your first antenatal visit on, or possibly before, this fictitious 'due date', is that the midwife will say, 'We induce at term plus ten days. We don't allow you to go beyond ten days' – and she will make an appointment for your induction in a week or ten days' time. If there is a particular clinical indication, then an induction may be justified, although the sensible thing to do is to ask questions about this and request the evidence and research to back it up, but the word 'allow' is not sufficient justification. It may be a good idea to also consult someone who has knowledge and experience but is not subject to hospital protocols. It is a mother's decision whether to be induced. In any other sphere of medicine, treatment is proposed, discussed and it is up to the patient to decide whether they want to go down that path. Yet it seems that often a pregnant woman is not treated with this degree of respect.

Women are told that there is a higher risk of stillbirth after 42 weeks according to the Cochrane review. But Cochrane themselves say that much of the research on which this is based is out of date or of poor quality. A study from 1958, over half a century ago, is the 'evidence' of a rise in stillbirth after 40 weeks. The increase is often misquoted as 'double at 42 weeks' – as explained in Gail Hart's article 'A Timely Birth' (in *Midwifery Today*, Issue 72, 2004). Then there are the figures from the MBRRACE report that are published every year.

On the surface these would seem to show that the percentage of stillbirths decreases after 42 weeks. But it is important to remember that this is an audit and not set up as research. We do not know, for example, whether these labours were induced or spontaneous, nor is there a control group for comparison. So it is difficult to get an accurate figure on which you can base your decision, but we do know that there is a considerable amount of fear-mongering and coercion that goes on to pressurise a woman into agreeing to an induction of labour, which is a significant intervention. In effect it is difficult to find up-to-date and accurate figures, although this is sometimes not the impression given to women when an induction is proposed.

An unofficial guesstimate is that fewer than 10 per cent of women go into labour spontaneously as 90 per cent agree to a sweep or a more medicalised induction. A sweep, it is important to remember, is also an induction of labour, as well as the more medicalised procedure.

A pregnant woman will not infrequently be asked, 'Don't you want to do the best for your baby?' And it is not unusual for a mother to report that she was asked, 'Do you realise your baby is twice as likely to die?' Coercion like this is illegal.

The law states that no procedure can be done without informed consent. The role of a caregiver is to give the information, risks and benefits of a procedure and the risks and benefits of not doing it. The mother then is in a position to make an informed choice, and it is the role of her caregivers to support her in that choice, regardless of their personal opinion. I mention this now because I would like you to think about this seriously, inform yourself, and make your choice.

It is impossible for you to understand the degree of pressure you will come under when you are 40 weeks pregnant and beyond, which it will for 85 per cent of you. Women have said to me, 'I never realised it would be like this.' So please think carefully, make your decision, and stick to it, unless there is a change in your clinical circumstances. If that happens, go back to the beginning and do your research.

You may have the first conversation with your midwife, who is then obliged to 'offer' an appointment with an obstetrician, though it doesn't feel like an offer to you. You feel that the obstetrician may have some additional important information to give you, and it would be irresponsible not to attend. You may have to wait some time, and then you may find that the obstetrician tells you exactly what the midwife has already said, but with more pressure. You may find yourself having the same conversation, and subjected to the same pressure, every time you go in for monitoring to check that your baby is fine.

You are within your rights to say that you heard and understood what you were told the first time, that you decline to have the offer made to you again, and ask to have this decision recorded in your notes so the conversation doesn't take place again.

You will, of course, as a responsible and intelligent parent, be open to having a new conversation if your clinical circumstances should change (and that doesn't mean because your pregnancy has extended another week), and it is important to remember, too, that many clinicians will simply give you a gentle and full explanation and leave it at that. However many women will agree to an induction by membrane sweep or even a medicalised induction, not because they want one, but simply because they can no longer stand the pressure that is being applied and to 'please' their caregivers.

Pressure like this simply puts you under stress. When you are stressed you are in the fear response. You cannot be in the fear response and the confident response at the same time. In the confident response you produce oxytocin and are more likely to go into labour. The more pressure that is heaped on you, the less likely you are to go into labour. It seems that the maternity system you find yourself in is designed to subject you to more and more pressure and stress with the threat of a sweep (a less medicalised induction) or an induction which actually, after 40 weeks, creates the situation of a longer pregnancy when an induction is supposed to be needed. Crazy world!

I am told that many women are told their placenta will fail, but I have heard of no evidence that this happens caused by length of pregnancy.

*'Placental insufficiency is an assumption that has never been proven. It is a theory based on nothing more than opinion and speculation, and there is no evidence to support it.'*
Wickham (2018)

*'It is known that infants born later in pregnancy have lower rates of special school needs.'*
Maiti et al (2017)

It can make sense to be monitored regularly beyond 42 weeks, to make sure all is well with your baby, and possibly even more to reassure you and give you confidence. This is clearly stated in the NICE guidelines. As ever, it is your choice. Mothers are also often told that their baby will grow too big to be born normally if it stays in the womb 'too long'. But some midwives say that a big baby can be born more easily as its head fills the pelvis and the uniform pressure of its head on the cervix efficiently stimulates the production of the hormones that assist the progress of labour. An ultrasound estimate of the size of the baby is only 80 per cent accurate, which is the difference between an 8lb and a 10lb baby. No-one really knows the size of a baby until it is born and weighed. The position and relaxation of the mother are by far the most important aspects to facilitate a straightforward birth.

The NICE guidelines specifically advise that induction is inappropriate for a big or little baby.

It is often normal and healthy for a baby to be born outside the 37–42 week period. It is a perfectly viable option to monitor the mother and baby beyond 42 weeks to make sure both are healthy and well and the pregnancy is progressing normally. If all is well, what's the rush? The choice to wait and be monitored may not be presented to you, so you may have to ask for it, but it can often be the safe and sensible route to take.

You could take the view that there is no such thing as a 'late baby'. It's simply that some women naturally have a different length pregnancy than others. If you're one of the lucky ones to experience a longer pregnancy, then feel blessed and enjoy this special bonus time!

On the pages that follow, you will find an additional script that will help you to rise above any pressure or coercion you may experience from well-meaning friends, family or your healthcare professionals. Use it if you need to: it will help you to remain calm and enjoy the bonus time in the last days and weeks of your pregnancy.

## *THE GIFT OF BONUS TIME RELAXATION*

Take three long, slow gentle breaths. Breathing in through the nose and out through the mouth. And on the out breath say to yourself **release, release, release**.

Now just imagine you are having a wonderful, calming massage with warm natural oils, and the lightest relaxing scent of lavender. With the first stroke up your back your realise you had not known how stressed you were until those stresses started to drop away and you begin to sink deeply into **calm and content**.

With the second stroke up your back you had never known such deep release, and you sink even more deeply into **comfort and wellbeing**.

With the third stroke up your back of this warm, sweet smelling, oil you sink into **ultimate peace, deep peace**.

When that wonderful massage comes to a close, you wrap yourself in a warm, soft robe and move to the recliner offered to you in a beautiful calm and quiet room. All is well as you enjoy the occasional kick inside you telling you that your baby is there with you, and relish the experience of being pregnant, looking forward positively and confidently to your baby's birth.

But then someone else comes into the room and asks you your due date. 'I don't have one,' you reply. 'Baby knows best.' 'Aren't you fed up with being pregnant so long?' they ask. 'Isn't it risky?' Now doubts begin to enter your mind. You begin to feel stressed that all may not be well. That wonderful feeling of confidence and trust is shaken a little. Then a little kick inside you seems to say, 'I'm here. All is well.' It reminds you of the special bonus you have been given of these last few days and weeks of pregnancy to enjoy, and you smile. The confidence returns, and you notice that the person who had intruded on your peace of mind has simply vanished. You take three long, slow breaths and you say to yourself, **Happy, positive, trust**.

You settle yourself comfortably on your recliner again in your warm, soft robe, and enjoy that wonderful feeling of wellbeing.

Someone else comes into the room now, to check that you are comfortable. 'Why haven't you had a sweep yet?' they ask. 'I decided not to,' you reply. 'But why not?' they press. You begin to have doubts and feel unsure. But then a tiny kick inside you brings you back to reality and you reply. 'What is the reason that you suggest it? It's up to you to give a reason if you want to interfere with my healthy pregnancy. I'm enjoying this special time, my bonus time.' When you finish speaking you realise that your questioner has disappeared, just melted away. The seeds of doubt that they tried to sow in your mind have disappeared too. You take three long, slow breaths as you say to yourself, **Confidence, calm, comfort**.

You settle back on your recliner again in your warm, soft robe. Your baby's gentle kick says to you, 'I'm here. I'm here,' and you relish this extra bonus time that you have been given.

Now someone else enters the room. 'Think what might happen to your baby in the next few days and weeks if you don't agree to an induction,' they say. The biggest fear of all enters your heart, fear for your baby's welfare. 'Think what might have happened to my baby throughout my pregnancy, but it didn't,' you respond. 'Tell my why it is likely to happen now. Show me the research. Give me good, up-to-date, accurate figures,' you reply. The effort of this conversation has

*Continued overleaf...*

*... Continued from page 183*

disturbed your peace of mind. You begin to doubt yourself. The doubt undermines your confidence and positivity. You felt so happy before, but now you feel stressed and the coercion and pressure is beginning to gnaw away at your confidence and positivity. You make a supreme effort to invoke again the happiness of this special bonus time, and you take three long, slow breaths. With each breath you generate oxytocin, the hormone or calm, the hormone of love, which permeates your very being, and you say to yourself, **Confidence, positivity, empowerment**.

As you look round you realise that this last person who tried to disturb your peace of mind has disappeared completely. Relief washes over you as you settle comfortably on your recliner in your soft, warm robe again. A gentle kick brings a smile to your face.

One more person comes into the room. This person moves calmly and gently. They sit down quietly beside you and you enjoy the comfort of their presence. They gently stroke your forehead, and any remaining stresses in your mind fade away. As your mind becomes calm and at ease again, utterly calm and positive, so your body sinks into ultimate peace. 'You have been given the privilege of carrying your baby inside you for a few extra days and weeks. This is bonus time, a time to be enjoyed and relished. A very special short extra time of togetherness. I will always be there for you, I will stay with you and protect you from any pressure or negative thoughts until your baby decides it is time to be born.'

As you snuggle into your warm soft robe again, and settle back on your recliner, you know that feeling of confidence and wellbeing is always there for you. Every time you feel a gentle kick it reinforces your positive assurance.

This feeling is always there for you. You are strong, and positive, and confident. This feeling will remain with you and grow every day for the whole of your pregnancy of whatever length. Your wonderful, special pregnancy.

Spend a few minutes enjoying this state of calmness and confidence and then:

Begin to notice the sounds around you.

Notice your eyelids beginning to flutter.

Gently open your eyes and come back to the present

Bringing the calmness and confidence with you.

## *Takeaways*

* The notion of a 'due date' is a harmful fallacy, putting pressure on you to consent to 'speeding up' the process once that date has passed.
* Consider pregnancy after 40 weeks as precious and important.
* Resist the tendency to give in to self-imposed stress after 40 weeks. Your baby will come when it is ready.
* Avoid stress after 40 weeks from your family and friends by not telling people your 'due date' or by adding two weeks to the date given to you and publicising that instead.
* Be informed of the facts about induction of labour either by sweep or by more medicalised procedures after about 40 weeks. Being well informed is important when you are subjected to pressure and coercion to persuade you to agree.
* Remain calm, confident and positive.

'Induction of labour, whether
medical or non-medical,
is always an attempt to
persuade your body to go
into labour before your baby
is ready to be born.'

Nadia Higson

'In an analysis of nearly 45,000
women who gave birth at term
in Brisbane, Australia, induction
was associated with a lower
chance of vaginal birth and a
higher chance of Caesarean
without better outcomes
for babies.'

Zhao et al (2017)

# CHAPTER 13

# Induction of Labour

## Induction by membrane sweep

This may already be written in your notes simply as 'sweep membranes', to take place at the first antenatal visit on or after your 'due date', or sometimes even before it. Your notes may say 'discuss membrane sweep', but a membrane sweep is so routine it is assumed it will happen. It is such a routine procedure that it is hardly considered an intervention; but it is an intervention – it is an induction under a different name. And no intervention should be done without informed consent. Many women are asking for a sweep from 37 weeks or even earlier, but they are probably not well informed, unlike you, because you have read this book. A membrane sweep is a significant intervention so you need to be well informed and consider carefully if you want to agree.

A membrane sweep consists of a midwife or obstetrician inserting two fingers into the cervix during a vaginal examination and 'sweeping' those two fingers round the cervix to try to lift the membranes off the cervix and massage the cervix to simulate what a baby's head would do to trigger labour. This can trigger the release of prostaglandins, which soften the cervix and can stimulate the onset of labour. To be thorough, a sweep should take about five minutes, and can be uncomfortable. If your body is nearly ready to go into labour, a sweep may be successful, but since your body was ready to go into labour soon anyway, what's the point? 'If we do a sweep today, it will save you from an induction next week, because baby will probably arrive quite quickly.' This is often quoted as justification for a sweep. If you think for a moment, this is not a rational argument, because the baby may have arrived by next week anyway, and if it hasn't you could decide to have a sweep then.

Before doing a sweep, a midwife will assess whether it is likely to be successful by using the Bishop score. This is an assessment of how nearly your body is ready to give birth, and your baby is ready to be born. The midwife will assess:

■ **Dilation of your cervix** Whether it has started to open, and if so, by how much.

■ **Effacement of your cervix** The cervix in pregnancy is about 3cm long, and it gradually becomes shorter and thinner as labour progresses.

■ **Consistency of your cervix** Normally your cervix is quite firm, like the cartilage on the end of your nose. As your body prepares to give birth it will become much softer like your ear lobe or your lip.

■ **Position of your cervix** The cervix is normally tucked up at the back of your vagina facing backward. As labour approaches it will turn forwards in the direction of the baby's way out.

■ **Foetal station** This means how far down your baby's head is in your pelvis.

If the Bishop score is 8 or above, your labour is likely to start soon as your body has already made the changes to indicate this, so why agree to an induction (by sweep or medicalised)? Your body is likely to go into labour soon spontaneously anyway.

If your Bishop score is low, your body has not begun to move towards giving birth, it would be difficult and uncomfortable if not painful to do a sweep as the cervix is still firm, inaccessible at the back of the vagina and closed, and the baby's head has not moved down into the pelvis where it applies pressure on the inside of the cervix to stimulate the hormones of birth. In these circumstances an induction by sweep, even if possible, is not likely to be effective, so why agree to it? A medicalised induction is likely to take a long time as your body is not ready, so why agree to it?

If there is a particular clinical indication for induction, that is a completely different situation, and is not what we are discussing here.

The outcome of a sweep is similar to the outcome of a medicalised induction of labour in terms of assisted deliveries and c-sections, so it has implications. One in eight sweeps are said to be successful insofar as you go into labour within 48 hours, but we don't know how many of these women would have gone into labour within 48 hours anyway. If it is not 'successful' you may have cramping that prevents you resting at night and then stops, and increases your levels of stress. When you do go into labour spontaneously you would be tired from lack of sleep and then this may affect the labour.

I have often heard of women who had a sweep, went into labour, and had a very long labour, and then wondered afterwards if the baby would have arrived at the same time but with a shorter labour if they had trusted it to come when it was ready.

## Medicalised induction of labour

Most labours in the UK are induced, either by a membrane sweep or a medicalised induction. For first-time mums, the medicalised induction rate is probably about 40 per cent. Of these, some midwives have told me that about 70 per cent are probably for 'post dates'. Some hospitals are beginning to put the 'post dates' inductions into different categories so they are given a different name. The rate varies from country to country, but the percentage is high, and the World Health

Organization is concerned at the level of medicalisation of birth. Consider this for a moment. For 40 weeks your baby has grown perfectly normally. You go to antenatal visits to make sure all is well but, in general, everyone has assumed that the mother and baby know the best way to grow a baby. Then you get to the fictitious 'due date', which we have already seen is based on poor mathematics, and everyone knows better than that baby what it should be doing. How can it be that so many mothers and babies have got it wrong?

Sometimes, when you attend your 40-week antenatal appointment, a midwife will make an appointment for your induction at 41.5 weeks. If this appointment is made, it will be hanging over you subconsciously and will subject you to low-level stress. To reiterate yet again, when you are stressed you are in the emergency response. You cannot be in the emergency response and the calm response at the same time. When you are in the calm response, you produce oxytocin, the hormone that facilitates labour, so the more stress you are put under the less likely you are to go into labour spontaneously.

Induction of labour is usually carried out in the labour ward rather than the birth centre as there is a greater likelihood of a need for further medical intervention. Labour will not start until the cervix has softened, as the muscle needs to relax and release, so the first procedure in a medicalised induction is to apply prostaglandin gel to soften the cervix. This is often applied in the form of a pessary which is rather like a tampon as this could be removed in the event of over-stimulation of the uterus. The tiny risk of this procedure is uterine rupture. It is interesting to note that this is not often mentioned to women. The risk of uterine rupture is mentioned to women who want a vaginal birth after a Caesarean (VBAC) but, in fact, the risk of a uterine rupture in this situation is actually less than when using a pessary to soften the cervix. Both risks are tiny, but it is interesting that the risk is mentioned when the woman is asking for normality but not mentioned when a medical intervention is being proposed. I stress that the risk is tiny in both cases.

A balloon catheter can also be used instead of the prostaglandin. This is a small soft plastic balloon that can be inserted into the cervix and then filled with saline. Again, the purpose is to stimulate the cervix and produce prostaglandin. The risk is that it lifts the baby's head off the cervix, which could allow space for the cord to slip down below the baby's head (cord prolapse) so the cord which supplies oxygen to the baby could become compressed during the birth process. Also, by lifting the baby's head off the cervix where it has settled ready for birth, the baby may descend into a less natural position which could have repercussions during the birth. As the balloon catheter has become more frequently used recently the risks and benefits are not yet well researched.

Sometimes using prostaglandin to soften the cervix is sufficient for labour to proceed but, since an induction by definition is done when labour has not started spontaneously, it is usual for the next step to follow. This involves the midwife reaching in through the cervix with an amniohook to break the membranes around the amniotic fluid. Once this has been done there is a risk of infection as the baby is no longer in a sealed unit, so the usual procedure is for the surges to be started artificially.

This is done with the use of synthetic oxytocin (generally referred to as Oxytocin in the UK or Pitocin in the USA). Either of these drugs is a synthetic form of oxytocin.

The staff will insert a cannula, a small plastic tube (guided in with a needle which is then removed), usually in the mother's hand or arm. The cannula is attached to a bag of fluid containing the synthetic oxytocin.

Natural oxytocin is pulsed into the body from the pituitary gland. The build-up and reduction are gradual: a wave-like movement. The natural oxytocin triggers the release of endorphins, nature's pain-relief, so, as labour becomes more efficient and intense, nature has provided the hormone to deal with this.

Surges that are artificially stimulated tend to start more abruptly and be more frequent, more painful and closer together. The synthetic oxytocin which is inserted straight into the circulation system does not cross the blood-brain barrier so does not stimulate the production of endorphins.

In a natural labour, the muscles of the uterus revert to a resting state between surges. In an induced labour, the muscles remain in a low state of tension and never completely rest, so there is a greater strain on the mother's body and on the baby.

In order to monitor how the more powerful surges that are induced artificially are affecting the baby, a CTG machine is attached to your abdomen to monitor your baby's heart. Attention now tends to be focused on the monitor rather than on you. A machine may give accurate information, but it still takes a human being to interpret that information and this interpretation can vary considerably from person to person.

You are now probably attached to two lines: the canula for the synthetic oxytocin and the monitor for the baby's heart which means you can't get into water as you are attached to electricity, so a birthing pool is no longer an option for you. It also means you cannot move around freely so it is harder to get into a position that is conducive to a more efficient and comfortable labour, though it can still be achieved with help from your partner.

An induced labour also means that you would have to be under the care of an obstetrician in a hospital obstetric unit, where more sophisticated emergency care is available. So you would be in a room with a bed and a chair, rather than at home or in a midwife-led unit (or birth centre), which is more likely to have rooms with birthing pools and birth balls, which generally encourage you to be in a position that could be more comfortable. You can kneel on a hospital bed with pillows on the sloping bed head, or sit on a birth ball beside the bed leaning forward on a pile of pillows.

Some hospitals have remote monitoring (telemetry) which makes movement easier and choice of position more flexible. Some hospitals will also facilitate the use of a birthing pool and make arrangements for the canula to have waterproof protection.

An induced labour is a much more intense experience than a labour that starts spontaneously; it is more intense for the mother and more intense for the baby, so there is more likely to be foetal distress. However, I have known mothers do the whole of an induced labour without needing drugs using their KGH techniques, which is a huge accolade for the mothers and for hypnobirthing – and also for her birth companion who is supporting her.

It is generally, however, a completely different experience from spontaneous labour.

The current NICE (National Institute for Clinical Excellence) says of induction:

> 'Induction of labour has a large impact on the health of women and their babies and so needs to be clinically justified.
>
> From 42 weeks, women who decline induction of labour should be offered increased antenatal monitoring consisting of at least twice-weekly cardiotocography (monitoring the baby's heart rate) and ultrasound estimation of maximum amniotic pool depth.'

It is up to a mother to choose, carefully considering medical advice, if she considers that being 41.5 weeks pregnant is a sufficiently 'clear clinical justification' for submitting herself to a procedure that has a 'large impact' on her health and the health of her baby (as quoted from the guidelines). The definition of 'clinical' from Webster's dictionary is, 'Based on or characterised by observable and diagnosable symptoms.' This is a very important decision as it can have profound repercussions, in terms of the comfort and ease of labour, how her birthing proceeds, the medical interventions that are performed, and how her baby enters the world. It is worth noting that an induction is always done in an obstetric unit rather than a birth centre because obstetric interventions are more likely.

The actual procedure of induction is not so very significant, but the repercussions of an induction should be considered very seriously. Throughout the induction there are likely to be many vaginal examinations to check on progress, and inserting anything into the vagina carries with it the risk of infection. Two things can happen as a result of an induction. If the baby was almost ready to be born anyway, the labour can be intense but quite short. If the baby was not ready to be born or the mother is stressed and fearful, then the labour can be long, and there will come a point when she will probably need a rest. The only way she can achieve this is by being given an epidural. An epidural is a sophisticated form of analgesia administered by an anaesthetist, who inserts a tube into the lower back through which drugs are injected via an attached catheter. The drugs block the transmission of nerve signals to the brain. You can have a light epidural (a walking epidural) which may have largely worn off before the actual birth of your baby and which can make it possible for you to walk. You can also have an epidural that you can top up yourself as needed but which also prevents you from overdosing. Because the epidural prevents sensations from your body reaching your brain, you will also be fitted with a catheter as you won't be able to feel when you need to empty your bladder.

You are now attached to four lines, the canula in your arm for the synthetic oxytocin, the monitor on your abdomen to listen to your baby's heart, the line for the epidural in your back, and the catheter to allow you to empty your bladder. You can see that things have changed very considerably from the natural birth you had planned, and you need to take all this carefully into account before you choose whether an induction is right for you and your baby. I'm telling you all this here because you may not get the information anywhere else.

The effect of the epidural is to slow things down, so it can slow down the surges and also the baby's heart. The strength of the synthetic oxytocin will then be increased to maintain the strength of the surges and you will not feel this because of the analgaesia. But the more powerful surges put more pressure on the baby which is why the baby's heart is being monitored. If the heartbeat slows, the baby is diagnosed as being in distress and a Caesarean section is suggested as the safest option.

Because the Caesarean has been agreed, the induction will not proceed so you will be taken off the synthetic oxytocin drip and surges may slow down or even stop as they had been artificially induced and were not being generated by your own body. It then might be some time before the Caesarean actually happens because the team has to be gathered in theatre. The anaesthetist, who is needed for the spinal block, may be in another theatre or placing an epidural for another woman. There is some dispute about the Caesarean level after an induction, but it seems that it is probably about twice the rate for a spontaneous labour.

An epidural is a sophisticated form of analgaesia, and anaesthetists are very skilled at what they do. They will do their best to administer an epidural that will largely have worn off before it is time for you to actually give birth to your baby. But no-one can foretell the length of labour, so the epidural block will still at least partly be in place and resulting in a lack of sensation, so the mother may not be able to feel when she needs to bear down.

As she cannot feel when to push, someone will need to coach her through this stage of labour rather than feeling her natural urge to expel her baby, which can be less efficient than her body telling her what to do, so she is more likely to need help to give birth to her baby in the form of forceps or ventouse. An episiotomy is usually performed when forceps are used which will need to be sutured after the birth and can lead to more bleeding.

In her book *Breech Birth* (2003), Benna Waites tells us that the use of an epidural results in a three-times increase in instrumental delivery, a significant increase in the length of the second stage of labour (when the mother bears down and the baby is born), and double the Caesarean rate.

We are very fortunate indeed to live in a society where interventions such as these are available when necessary, but there is a very big question about the over-medicalisation of birth, and the routine use of interventions which may not always be appropriate.

I would like to tell you a story that relates to inductions. When I was expecting my fourth baby I was planning to give birth at a small private hospital. I had no problem with the care I had received from the NHS; it was simply that during my pregnancy I had been looking after three little boys and I knew I was shortly going to be looking after three little boys and waking in the night to feed a new baby. So the concept of a room on my own for just a couple of days was extremely attractive.

My baby was due on 6 December, a Thursday. At the end of November I went for an antenatal appointment, and after the usual checks there was a sharp drawing in of breath, a bit like a builder looking at a house, and I was told that I needed to be induced on 4 December. Jargon and phrases like 'fourth baby' and 'much safer for the baby' were thrown at me, and if somebody says to a mother it is safer for her baby, she will agree to anything. The phrase was used in the past and it is used now. I pointed out that all my other babies had arrived two to four days so-called late, so plainly my natural length of pregnancy was about 40.5 weeks, which is perfectly normal. They said, 'No, it will be safer. We'll book you in for an induction on 4 December.'

So I went for my final antenatal visit on 3 December, but in the meantime my three sons had caught chicken pox. Other parents are generally quite prepared to look after children with chicken pox, since they would like their own children to get it, but not just before Christmas when Granny is about to come to stay and everybody wants to be a happy family. It is almost impossible to find someone to look after three little boys with chicken pox just before Christmas. So I went to my last visit before the scheduled induction saying, 'I don't think I can come to be induced on Tuesday because all my sons have chicken pox.' They looked at me in utter horror and said, 'Well, you can't have your baby here then.' A week before it had been very important that I should be induced for the safety of my baby, and a week later I was almost unceremoniously kicked out into the gutter. Remember this was a small private hospital and, if they had an epidemic of chicken pox, they couldn't have taken people in, they would have lost income and their reputation would have plummeted. Maybe they would even have had to close.

I went back to the NHS hospital where I had had my other babies. They took me in, there was no mention of an induction, I went into labour spontaneously, and my daughter was born without an induction on the afternoon of 8 December, two days so-called late just like her brothers. Better still, because of my sons' chicken pox, they put me in a little room on my own right at the end of the corridor, which I didn't have to pay for! Then they forgot me, which was wonderful, as I had four or five hours with my new baby completely undisturbed.

The real reason for the planned induction did not occur to me until I started to teach KGH. Then I received reports from lots of women planning to give birth at different midwife-led units and hospitals, and it gradually became clear that the reason they had wanted to induce me was to make sure my baby was not born at the weekend. It was the first weekend in December when there are lots of Christmas parties and people want to do their Christmas shopping. Maybe the consultant had a particular family gathering that he wanted to attend. Induce me on Tuesday, the baby is bound to have arrived by Friday, and everybody is happy – except mother and baby.

It is amazing the number of inductions that are done for convenience. It sounds very callous, but it is not entirely, because any hospital has a maternity unit to run. They have to think of their staff. They have to manage everything for the overall good, and there will be a great many inductions just before Christmas and just before Easter. Maybe if a lot of mothers are booked in to give birth the following week, they want to get through a few early so they can give the best possible care to everybody.

The birth rate increases around the full moon, so, if some women are induced the previous week, the staffing level for all can be managed more efficiently. Do bear this in mind and ask some questions if you are not quite sure why an induction is being suggested. Inductions are sometimes done at maternal request for the mother's convenience too.

## Circumstances where an induction might be suggested

There are some particular circumstances where an induction of labour may be suggested to a healthy woman other than for length of pregnancy. Here are a few of them:

■ **Older Mother** This means a woman who is 40 or older, and some hospitals take it as being 35 or older. In some cases (not all) there is a very slight increase in stillbirth with a longer pregnancy, but there is no research to show whether induction of labour reduces this risk.

■ **IVF Babies** There may be a very slight increased risk of still birth for IVF babies, but this may reduce as pregnancy progresses, and there is no research to indicate that induction of labour improves this situation.

■ **Twins** 60% of mothers carrying twins go into labour spontaneously before 37 weeks so the question of induction of labour does not arise. You would need to read more information than I can offer here, and the book below has an excellent section for twin mothers giving the research available.

You can find good information about induction in these and other circumstances in *The AIMS Guide to Induction of Labour* by Nadia Higson.

## Inducing labour more naturally?

Some people try to bring on labour themselves to avoid a medical induction. But please remember that this is still a form of induction; it is still saying to your baby that you know better than he or she does when is the right time for their birth. Here is a list of things people try.

■ **Lovemaking** Semen contains prostaglandins, which help to soften the cervix, and when you make love you relax and produce oxytocin, which stimulates uterine surges during labour, because you are in the parasympathetic nervous system. So there are two sound chemical reasons why making love could be a way to bring on labour, but only if the body is ready anyway.

One mother said to me, 'We have made love every day to try to make the baby come.' I did hope that this pressure wouldn't put them off making love for ever more.

The pressure to 'try to make the baby come' is sometimes because many birth centres will not admit a mother beyond 41.5 weeks or whatever is the rule in that hospital and after that she would be sent to delivery suite. You might like to get in touch with BirthRights (birthrights.org.uk) if you are told this as it cannot be substantiated legally. Until recently you still had the right to stay at home to give birth to your baby, but that right is being eroded too, although there may be greater flexibility about this choice. In fact, if you decided to stay at home to give birth and called a midwife, someone would have to come, even though you may have been told that they will not support you in this choice beyond 42 weeks. It is your right to be attended by a competent midwife wherever or whenever you give birth.

■ **Nipple and clitoral stimulation** Every midwife knows that this stimulation could possibly help bring on labour, though it is possibly more likely to start labour to get going again if the surges have slowed down, and some may suggest it. But why? Why not take the opportunity for a rest. If you ask for privacy to do this at home or in the hospital it is simply asking for something that everyone knows could work.

■ **Laughter** It's universally acknowledged that laughter relaxes you, and if a mother is relaxed she is more likely to go into labour because she is in the parasympathetic nervous system. It is an excellent idea, which I strongly recommend, to have list of half a dozen funny and light-hearted movies ready to use

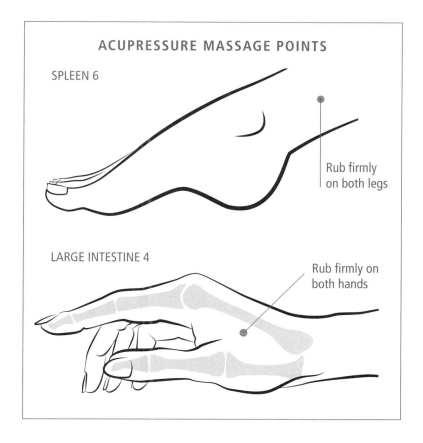

## ACUPRESSURE MASSAGE POINTS

SPLEEN 6

Rub firmly
on both legs

LARGE INTESTINE 4

Rub firmly on
both hands

for a stressful situation in late pregnancy or in early labour. Prepare your list now.

■ **Acupressure massage** See the illustrations on page 201 to help you to locate two acupressure points that can help.

Spleen 6 (Sp 6) – find and rub this point on both your legs: four finger-widths up the calf from the top back 'corner' of the inside ankle bone.

Large Intestine 4 (LI 4) – this point is found on the side of the bone of your index finger, near the junction with your thumb. Press very firmly in towards the underside of the bone.

■ **Hypnotherapy** This is the most effective complementary therapy. The body follows where the mind leads.

■ **Homoeopathy, aromatherapy, reflexology, acupuncture** A range of other complementary therapies can also be effective. Use these to achieve relaxation, not to 'make the baby come'.

■ **Visualising an opening rosebud** Picturing in your mind a soft and open image has a softening and opening effect on the body. It's simple and remarkably effective and the simple things are often best. Find a picture of a beautiful pink, full-blown rose and display it in your home from week 37. If you decide to go to hospital, take it with you. If you hold an image of soft and open in your mind, guess what your body is doing.

■ **Walking** Midwives often suggest this, but Michel Odent advises against it as walking produces adrenaline, which inhibits the production of oxytocin, the hormone that facilitates the working of the uterine muscles. You might enjoy a gentle stroll, but a brisk walk saps your energy – energy that you will need for giving birth to your baby.

■ **Taking a bath** This is another good way to relax, and relaxing always helps. You could add essential oil of lavender to the water, have night lights around the edge, and your

KGH audio playing in the background.

■ **Hot and spicy foods** Undoubtedly some women have gone into labour after a hot curry, but if it were that effective every woman in India would miscarry. Mainly an old wives' tale.

■ **Raspberry leaf tea** This is a muscle toner not directly related to triggering labour. Many women who have reached 40 weeks, and even before, drink raspberry leaf tea by the gallon. I would ask you to quietly consider why you are doing it and what is best for your baby

■ **Eating dates** This is the only item on this list that has been properly researched. The research was done in Jordan, a part of the world where delicious dates are grown and these are considered to be good for pregnant women to eat. The original research studied a group of pregnant women who ate 6 dates a day from week 36 and a group that did not. The result was only very small, but was replicated in subsequent trials. The date-eating group went into labour very slightly sooner, they were very slightly further dilated when they met their midwife, and the first stage of labour was slightly shorter.

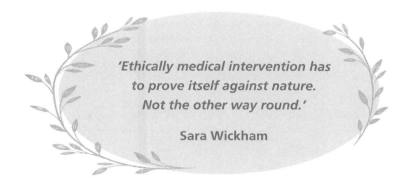

*'Ethically medical intervention has to prove itself against nature. Not the other way round.'*

**Sara Wickham**

If you are doing something to try to bring on labour, you are effectively saying to yourself that there is something wrong with the present situation. If you have decided there is something wrong, you have put yourself in a state of low-level stress. If you are in a state of stress, even at a low level, you are in the fear or emergency response, the sympathetic nervous system. As we saw in Chapter 2, you cannot be in the emergency response and the calm and confident response (the parasympathetic nervous system) at the same time. If you are in the calm and confident response, your body produces oxytocin, which is the hormone that stimulates the uterine muscles to work in labour, and therefore your baby is much more likely to put in an appearance. The body is inhibited from releasing your baby when you are in a state of fear, even low-level stress, if it can possibly help it.

## Takeaways

* Induction often leads to greater medical intervention during birth. It's most likely to work if the baby is ready to be born in any case.

* Induction by membrane sweep is practically routine, but remember, a sweep is still an induction.

* Medicalised induction is a significant intervention that can set in chain a whole sequence of potential implications, often called the cascade of interventions. Make sure you are well informed so you can make the right decisions for you.

* Many 'natural' induction procedures are either old wives' tales or based on relaxing, which will always help with preparing your body for birth. Some may have an effect. Most will not. But the idea 'trying to make your baby come' indicates stress. Stress triggers adrenaline, and adrenaline inhibits the production of oxytocin, and oxytocin is the hormone that facilitates labour.

# CHAPTER 14

# Asking Questions

When you hear the words 'allow', 'this is what we do' or 'we don't let you', I would suggest that you ask a few questions, because it is up to you whether you give consent, and you need full information in order to do so. Ask questions at any time that a procedure is suggested and you don't feel comfortable about it or you are not quite sure. It's your body and it's your baby. I'm not suggesting you simply tell a midwife or an obstetrician, 'No, I don't want that.' That would be rude and ill-informed; they have a great deal of knowledge and experience that should be respected but it is important that you are the leading member of the team and central to the decision-making process, which means you are also part of the dilemma that doctors and midwives face.

Healthcare professionals face dilemmas daily. They are subjected to guidelines that they don't necessarily agree with, and they have to deal with the bureaucracy of the NHS on a daily basis, as well as the politics and possibly even bullying within the department. It is seldom that anything is black and white, that 'This is the right thing to do, and that is wrong.' It is more often a case of 'Taking everything into account, I think this would be a good option to try first' – bearing in mind that doing nothing can often be the best choice of all.

No sensible person would object to any of the procedures suggested to help in certain medical circumstances. The problem arises when things are done routinely or frequently, sometimes without giving a full explanation, and without looking carefully at a woman's individual circumstances, and taking her views into account, as well as giving her the evidence and research for a proposed intervention.

Never allow yourself to be rushed into making a decision. These are important choices that can affect you for the rest of your life and your baby for the whole of its life. Remember the acronym F.A.S.T: Stand back and consider the facts.

F **Fear or Feeling** We'll think about Fear first. The brain cannot work properly to make a logical decision when we are afraid. We are in the fight/flight mode, and our blood supply is focused on supplying our arms and our legs efficiently.

But you could also say that F is for Feeling. Feeling is not a good basis for an important decision. Feeling may be just an idea that you have been brought up with, so you feel comfortable with it and uncomfortable with anything that threatens it. Feeling and instinct are completely different, but they are often confused. We will talk about instinct later. Make your decision based on evidence and logic.

A **Assumptions** As we have seen before, what we call decisions are often assumptions based on what 'everyone knows'. Make sure you come to real decisions. Evidence and logic apply here too.

S **Social pressure** 'You're mad to think of giving birth at home.' 'You can't have proper care unless you go to an obstetrician.' 'Hasn't your baby arrived yet?' 'Shouldn't you be induced by now?' 'Don't you want the best for your baby?' None of these statements are good reasons for agreeing to a major intervention, although it may be tempting at the time, simply to relieve the pressure.

T **Time** Never be rushed into making a decision. These choices are important. Always take your time.

I am certainly not advocating confrontation, that would be rude and unacceptable, but some polite questions can be very helpful in these circumstances:

## Useful questions

*I wonder if you can help me?*
This is a really effective question to use at the beginning of any conversation that could be difficult. Nobody would say, 'No.' They might not be able to say 'Yes', but they will almost certainly say something like, 'I'll do my best', and then you're both on the same side at the start of the conversation, which is always the best place to be.

*Could you explain that to me?*
This question is perfectly courteous and reasonable and is even quite complimentary, because it recognises that the person you are speaking with is an expert, which indeed they are. But you are entitled to an explanation, and if you get a good explanation all other questions are superfluous. Sadly, though, sometimes you don't.

I remember a woman expecting twins who asked me questions in a KGH class which were really medical questions, so I suggested she should ask her obstetrician. The answer her obstetrician gave was, 'Because we think it's best', which is hardly a rational explanation to give to an intelligent adult. It would be insulting and unacceptable to a two-year-old child.

*What other options are there that we could consider first?*
The staff in a busy maternity unit sometimes don't have time to explain everything to everybody although they do their best. Some are very good at it and some less so, but if you ask, there are almost always other options, and you are entitled to be told about them and consider them. You might have to go to someone outside the unit to get this question answered.

## How would what you're suggesting affect my labour (or my partner's labour)?

When I had my fourth baby I went into labour on a Saturday afternoon at about midday, and at four o'clock very little seemed to be happening and I was getting bored. My husband was even more bored. He was sitting on a stool beside me nodding off, so he went to the waiting room to find a more comfortable chair for a snooze. I remarked to the midwife that this labour was taking rather a long time. You might think that four hours is a reasonable length of time for labour, but my first baby had arrived in six hours, my second in two hours, my third in half an hour, and so four hours was a rather unacceptable length of time as far as I was concerned.

The midwife was very kind and suggested, 'Baby would arrive quite quickly if I broke your waters.' Then, it being England and four in the afternoon, she asked, 'Would you like a cup of tea first?' So I had a cup of tea at 4pm, they broke my waters at 4.10pm, and baby arrived at 4.20pm. That quickly. It was a very hard and fast ten minutes, of continuous powerful, very painful contractions and I would never have agreed had I had any idea what it was going to be like. Had it been my first baby it would have been absolutely devastating, and it was an experience I would never want to repeat. But nobody had said a word to explain the effects of the procedure, because it was so routine. Research shows that rupturing membranes (breaking waters) does not in fact make a significant difference to the length of labour, so please don't think having your waters broken will mean your baby will be born within ten minutes. Yes, I gave consent. No, I did not give informed consent because I hadn't been given any information on which to base my decision.

If we had asked my caregivers how their suggestion would affect labour, just possibly we might have been told that the surges are likely to be stronger and more painful. Then I could have made a more informed choice. And of course, if the surges are stronger and more painful for the mother, this is likely to put more pressure on the baby too.

**How would it affect the baby?**
This is also a very valid question – see above.

**What are the risks and possible negative outcomes of an induction of labour, particularly with an epidural?**
Possibly the biggest question of all, and one which many women wish they had asked after the event.

**Why do so many women report a traumatic birth?**
This is a growing epidemic and can be prevented if you are educated and take responsibility for your birth so you work as a team with your caregivers.

**Is it likely in this case?**
This question can be useful if a particular procedure is proposed to avoid some possible negative outcome. Many procedures are done prophylactically (preventively) to everyone to prevent harm in a tiny number of cases. You are entitled to be told the chance of that event happening so you can make up your own mind whether to agree to the procedure. It could be that the procedure is relevant to you – or maybe not.

**What will happen if we don't do this?**
Most people go into hospital when they are ill, for something to be done, and so doing something tends to be the default option of a hospital. But the option of not doing anything can be an extremely good one in many cases. Pregnant women

are the only people who go into hospital hoping that nothing will be done. Staying at home is most likely to achieve this. So often, baby knows best.

### Are you suggesting this because it's hospital protocol, or is it evidence based?

You must respect the fact that there are, quite rightly, guidelines and protocols, and it is very difficult for a midwife to go against these protocols. She has to tick boxes. She will be in trouble if she does not, and her career might be put in jeopardy. If there weren't guidelines, protocols and boxes to tick, things might get left out, and there would be chaos. However, remember that they should be guidelines, and not rules that are followed religiously whatever the circumstances. Guidelines are a checklist for the midwife of procedures she should offer you They are not rules that you have to follow. Ask your midwife. This gives her the space to talk around the issue, maybe a little more freely, rather than telling you simply, 'This is what we usually do.' In order not to tick the box, she has to be able to record that she offered you the procedure, and she has to cover herself and the hospital legally by writing 'mother declined' on your notes, and you need a sensible discussion of the facts in order to make that decision. The phrase, 'what you are asking is outside guidelines' is sometimes used, implying that you are putting your baby at risk. This is not necessarily the case. Only 12 per cent of the Royal College of Obstetrician and Gynaecologists' guidelines are based on grade A research. It is always appropriate to politely ask questions and make sure you have been given the full information and are confident that any proposed intervention is right for you and your baby. I know it can feel like a heavy responsibility, but it's the only way you will get the best possible birth experience. It is one of the roles of your birth partner to help you find out the information you need and protect you in this way.

***Please give me the evidence and research, so I have good information to make my choice.***
Of course, nobody can be absolutely sure of the outcome of an intervention, but if you can't be reasonably sure, why would you agree to it? It is certainly worth asking this question.

***I'm just going to record our conversation so I can consider the information you give me afterwards.***
You are legally entitled to record the conversation at a consultation. It can ensure that the conversation is rational with no emotional pressure.

The answers you are given sometimes turn out to be non-answers when you listen to them at home. Saying that what you plan is 'outside guidelines' is a non-answer, as is 'because of your age' or 'because of your BMI'. You need the evidence to justify these statements.

***Would you put that in writing, please?***
If your doctor tells you that you or your baby are at risk by not accepting a specific intervention. I am not suggesting that you should ask your unfortunate caregivers to write down what they say every time they open their mouths. But occasionally I hear reported to me something that has been said that is quite outrageous and frightening to a pregnant woman. In these circumstances, what would be written down would be more factual and less emotionally charged than what was said. That is the purpose of this question. After all, you are required to sign that you agree to a procedure such as a Caesarean section, so it would seem reasonable to ask the obstetrician to sign the reason why a procedure is proposed.

I often hear of enormous pressure being put on mothers to agree to proposed interventions, and reports of mothers being told things like 'Don't you want to do the best for your baby?' or sometimes even, 'Do you want your baby to die?' to frighten them into agreeing to a particular procedure. If you ask an obstetrician or midwife to put something in writing, they might possibly modify what they have been saying.

Remember, you cannot be in the sympathetic nervous system (the emergency response) and the parasympathetic nervous system (the calm, normal response) at the same time. You are in either one or the other. When you are under stress you are in the sympathetic nervous system. It's when you are in the parasympathetic nervous system, the calm normal response, that you produce oxytocin, the hormone that facilitates the working of the uterine muscles in labour, and endorphins, the hormone of comfort. The more stress that is heaped upon you, the less likely you are to go into labour. It is also impossible to make a rational decision when you are under stress.

While one woman I taught was in labour at 36 weeks, her husband suddenly said, 'I've got to get the questions', and rushed off to get them, because he felt he would support her better if he knew helpful questions to ask. You too may find these questions very useful and they should be borne in mind seriously. In the event, this mother gave birth to a baby who weighed over 6lb, a perfectly normal size, so it seems that her natural length of pregnancy was less than the average 37–42 weeks: an example of a healthy baby of normal size being born outside the average time parameters.

I'm not suggesting that you need to learn these questions to ask verbatim, but you will find it helpful to be thinking along these lines and making sure your questions are fully answered.

# B.R.A.I.N.S.

Remember that the law in the UK says no intervention may be done without informed consent. This includes informed refusal. You may wish to politely remind your caregivers of this. Some things are done so routinely that they forget they are interventions. Once you have carefully taken advice and made your decision, any further discussion can be regarded as harassment.

A useful acronym for decision-making is B-R-A-I-N-S:

**B** enefits
**R** epurcussions
**A** lternatives
**I** nformation
**N** othing
**S** mile

Each procedure has Benefits; each procedure has Repercussions or Risks – always. Being told the risks of doing nothing and the benefits of what is proposed is not a full explanation. Both courses of action have benefits, and both have risks. You are entitled to know the research and the statistics for both.

For example, if you want to do something as simple as crossing the road, the benefit is that you want to get to the other side, and the risk is that there is traffic coming. If you are on your own, you will make a completely different choice than you would if you were accompanied by a child. You are an intelligent adult and you can make your own choice, but be sure you have been told the risks and benefits in order to do this.

There are always Alternatives, and if they haven't been presented to you then you need to ask. I am not saying that the alternatives are necessarily best, but to be told you have no choice is seldom an accurate assessment of the situation.

The 'I' stands for Information. The whole purpose of the B.R.A.I.N.S. acronym is to remind you to make sure you have got the facts at your disposal before you make your decision. Do you have enough information to make a sensible choice? The letter 'N' is for Nothing. Nothing is a wonderful thing to do; it is much the best course of action until informed logic tells you that something else is an improvement.

The last letter, 'S', stands for Smile. Smiling makes you feel good and makes the person being smiled at feel good. It builds relationships, and is a great way of starting any meeting. Some people prefer to say that S stands for Statistics. If someone says to you, 'Do you realise x (some dreadful event) could happen?' it scares you. If you ask for the statistic and you find that the likelihood is 0.001 per cent it sounds a great deal less scary, and then you ask about adverse reactions which arise in, say, 0.24 per cent of cases, you are then in a position to give informed consent if you so choose. Without that information even if you did give your consent it would not be informed consent and therefore performing the procedure would be highly questionable.

There are many healthcare professionals who take great care to give full explanations to the women in their care. Sometimes there simply isn't the time and, in those cases, you need to step in and take responsibility.

Remember, **YOU CANNOT MAKE A GOOD DECISION WHEN YOU ARE STRESSED.**

In a situation like this you might need to ask some further questions. Never be rushed into making a decision. How often have you made a snap decision and regretted it? Maybe you have agreed to something as simple as going to see a movie one evening, then gone home and thought, 'I wish I hadn't agreed. I don't really want to see that film, and I would much rather stay at home and put my feet up.' When it comes to

## HOW TO RELIEVE STRESS

- Go home and take a few more 'up' breaths with a positive statement on the out breath such as 'calm' or 'thank you'.
- Ask your partner to read you one of the relaxations you have been practising or read one to yourself. I would suggest the *Confident & Positive* script would be appropriate.
- Make yourself a cup of tea or a cool drink.
- Sit with your feet up and watch one of the funny movies you have prepared.
- Then have a long relaxing warm bath, with essential oil of lavender in the water, candles round the edge, and your *Ultimate Birth Relaxation* audio playing in the background.
- While you are soaking in the bath, your devoted partner is preparing the most delicious meal, or booking at your favourite restaurant, or ordering a superb takeaway.
- You sit down and have a romantic, candle-lit dinner for two.
- You may like to have half a glass of wine as a little treat at this dinner. I am completely against alcohol in pregnancy as it is known to affect the growth of your baby. If you have now reached, say, 41 weeks, your baby is fully developed and, if you go into hospital to be induced, the drugs that are used may be heroin derivatives that are far more harmful than half a glass of wine which might help you chill and go into labour spontaneously. Many midwives will suggest this, but no-one would write it down!
- Do your normal evening practice:
- Up breathing with visualisations
- Reading a relaxation. From week 40 onwards you might like to choose the *Confident & Positive* script more frequently.
- Turn on the audio
- Go to sleep

You will then have a relaxing night's sleep and, when you wake in the morning, you will feel refreshed, your mind will be clear, and you and your partner can sit down together and decide what you would like to do.

Then convey your decision to your caregivers.

NEVER MAKE A DECISION FROM A STATE OF FEAR.

your baby's birth, these are very important decisions. Always take your time. Say, 'Thank you for your advice, but we need a little time to think about what you've just told us.' Take a few 'up' breaths with a positive statement on the out breath such as 'calm' or 'thank you'.

---

## INSTINCT

I cannot over-emphasise the importance of instinct as the over-arching principle to apply when you are giving birth. Yes, find facts first. Yes, do the research. Yes, make rational decisions. But, having done all that, trust your instinct as a mother. You are the only true authority in the birthing room as you are the person giving birth. Everyone else is simply there in case you would like support. They are wonderful people and you respect their knowledge and experience, but you work together as a team, and you are the leader of the team.

Once your baby is born, you will be responsible for caring for it and making decisions about it. Take responsibility now to achieve the birth you want and, if something doesn't feel right, don't do it. Trust your INSTINCT.

---

## Objective medical advice

I strongly recommend that, if you have a dilemma over a medical issue, it would be worth making an appointment with an independent midwife for some objective, experienced advice; just an hour will do. Arrange either a face-to-face appointment or a virtual appointment to talk it through, and you will find that you definitely receive good, objective information, and it will clear your head and help to put your mind at rest. A telephone consultation may be the most practical solution. She has the same training and knowledge as NHS midwives, but she is free from the protocols of an individual hospital and so can take a more objective view. She also often has more experience of less usual circumstances as many women have turned to her in this situation whereas, in the NHS, these women would have been referred to an obstetrician and become a statistic in the epidemic of inductions that is happening these days, or else would have had a Caesarean. You can find a list of independent midwives at www.imuk.org.uk. The AIMS helpline is also extremely helpful: 0300 365 0663.

# Takeaways

* Ask questions and make sure the answer is evidence-based or logical. 'This is what we do' won't do.

* Remember the F.A.S.T. acronym to make sure that you never make a decision out of fear.

* Familiarise yourself with some useful questions so that you know what to ask.

* Use the B.R.A.I.N.S. procedure for making a decision that is calm and well-informed.

* Take time to relax and think clearly. Don't be rushed into a decision if you are stressed.

* An independent midwife can offer objective, experienced advice if you need support.

* Trust your instincts. As your baby's mother, your caregivers are there to support you.

* Use the *Confident and Positive* fear release relaxation to settle you when you have a difficult decision to make or just need to calm any fears you may have.

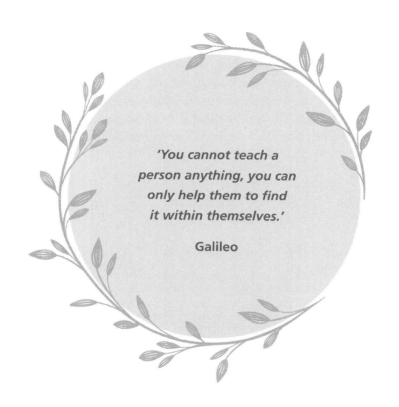

'You cannot teach a
person anything, you can
only help them to find
it within themselves.'

Galileo

CHAPTER 15

# Releasing Fear and Building Confidence

The very effective script on the following pages will help you to release fears and build confidence ready for the birth of your baby. Take your time over it and find an especially quiet time. Ask your partner to read it to you or read it to yourself, either silently or out loud.

You can also get the audio, *Confident and Positive*, if you prefer to listen to it together.

## When to use this script

This is not a relaxation and release for everyday practice, but to be used if something happens that gives you a major wobble: maybe you hear a very negative birth story, or something happens that you hadn't foreseen. Then take out this script and use it again, so you can deal with that circumstance, or anything else that may arise.

It's a special tool for a particular occasion. I know that some people like this script so much that they also include it from time to time in their daily practice.

There are two particular occasions to use this script:

▧ Use it as the script in your daily practice after Week 40 to relieve the stress that will be heaped on you at this time by your friends and caregivers (hopefully you will have dealt with your own stress by using the information in this book).

▧ At the beginning of labour. It is a great way to establish a calm and positive mindset.

## CONFIDENT AND POSITIVE RELAXATION

Sit comfortably or lie down completely at ease and take three long, slow, easy breaths. Now allow your eyes to close, slowly and gently. Just release, soften, release. Notice your breathing, how soft and quiet it has become, as you release even further.

**Now** you may begin to feel just as peaceful throughout your entire body, so you allow a wave of warmth and content to wash all through you, starting at the very top of your head as a gentle, warm, golden light that flows softly through every part of you. Slowly it moves down through your head, your eyelids, all around your eyes, your cheeks, your lips, your jaws.

Everything calms and releases. Just let that golden warmth spread on down through your neck, your shoulders, and down your arms. Now it flows down into your chest, through your stomach, the warm gentleness runs down your back, through your pelvis, all the way down your legs, your upper legs, your knees, your lower legs, your feet, until it reaches your toes, and every single part of your body is completely calm in this gentle golden glow.

Everything around you helps you to release more and more deeply, your breathing, the music, my quiet voice. Even if an unexpected sound breaks in, like traffic passing outside, or voices, or a phone ringing, that sound will simply prompt you to release even more, and you focus on my voice.

**Now** just imagine yourself at the top of a wide and shallow staircase with ten steps leading downwards. This is a very safe staircase with wide, shallow steps and it feels very attractive to you, so you begin to walk down. And as you walk down you count the steps ...

**Ten** Your foot goes safely down onto the first step and you have just started on your way down, gently and easily ...

**Nine** You find yourself going deeper into peace and wellbeing as you take the next step down, going deeper with it ...

**Eight** As you take the next step down, you go further into yourself ....

**Seven** Your whole body starts to feel completely weightless ...

**Six** You are floating on a wave of calm and serenity as if on a soft cloud ...

**Five** Deeper, deeper still ...

**Four** You have entered your own true self, deeply and willingly ...

**Three** You are so focused within your whole being that nothing touches you but your own true self, your wisdom, your intuition.

**Two** Everything is slipping away but your mind and your thoughts ...

**One** You feel completely, deeply and wonderfully calm, free of all care and worries, happy and peaceful. Even your thoughts are fading into oblivion. So deep; so very, very deep ...

**Rest**. Just rest happy and peaceful for a while: there's plenty of time ...

*(Continue with the pauses indicated above)*

**Now** imagine a blue-skied summer's day and you are lying on soft, dry grass under a tree by the sea. A warm, gentle

*Continued overleaf...*

*... Continued from page 221*

breeze just lightly touches your cheek. You are completely serene, happy and peaceful. As you look up, you notice that the leaves of the tree have pictures of all your happy memories, all the good things in your life, but also a few of them have images of the upsetting things in your life, and the things that make you wonder about giving birth. As you look at the leaves you notice some images that bring to mind things you have heard or read or thought about the concerns of childbirth, or perhaps your own previous experience of giving birth. As you observe and study the first one, you notice that the image gradually fades into the leaf itself which then turns yellow, brown, then gold – the colours of autumn – meaning the leaf has come to the end of its time, and neither it nor the thought it held matter any longer; and then the leaf just drops off the tree and lands beneath it.

**Now** you notice another leaf with another stress or worry and it too gently fades and dissolves into the leaf which changes colour and flutters to the ground, joining the first one. As you look, each time a fear you have comes to mind, a leaf takes on that image, which then fades and disappears as the leaf changes colour and falls to earth.

You realise now that you are able to see any stresses in the leaves, so you just take all the time you need to make sure all are dealt with – worries about birth, or anything else that comes to mind that you would like to easily release – and you find that one by one the same thing happens. The image of each concern is taken on by a leaf, and is absorbed right into the leaf, until it completely disappears. And all the leaves concerned change colour through the shades of autumn – yellow, gold, brown – and flutter to earth, taking their now vanished stresses and worries with them, and when the process is complete you sweep the leaves up into a heap.

**Now** only happy and positive green leaves are left on the tree and as you wonder what to do with the pile of leaves beside you, you have an idea. You decide you will have a bonfire, and invite to it all the people who have helped you in the past, or who are helping you now, or who are going to help you at this wonderful and important time in your life. Soon they start to arrive. They all come. You're both there of course, your loved ones, friends from throughout your life including right back to school, perhaps some of the people who taught you, your midwife, doctor, employers, colleagues, neighbours, just everyone who has ever helped or supported you, and those who will support you during the rest of your pregnancy and your baby's birth.

When they have all arrived and you are one big happy gathering, you set light to the bonfire, and it blazes quickly, and the leaves that had all the upsetting memories start to burn and curl up in the crackling flames. As they curl up and burn they turn to ash, and the ash rises in the heat and, as it rises, the gentle breeze picks it up and wafts it out to sea. You watch as it floats further and further out over the water, until it completely vanishes from sight, and as it vanishes completely, those memories and feelings the leaves carried vanish completely with it, gone forever, leaving you so confident and calm, peaceful and happy.

You feel so confident as you realise you now completely accept yourself, and accept your intuitive power to control your own life and look after yourself and your baby. Although all these people have helped or are helping you or will help you,

*Continued overleaf...*

*... Continued from page 223*

you now see that, while you may choose to accept their help, gladly and gratefully, you remain in control of your own life, and you and only you decide how things are to be, and how they may help you so that your baby is born so easily and happily, entering the world in the best possible way and giving you an empowering and joyful experience. And with this wonderful self-confidence and happiness, your guests slowly fade away, and leave you to your new self, knowing you can call them whenever you want them, and you will know when and how their wisdom, experience and knowledge may help you.

These thoughts lead you to realise that you can decide how you want the birth of your baby to be. You decide how your labour is, just how short a time it takes. Will it be less than 8 hours, 5 hours, 3 hours? Take a little while now to choose. Consider too how comfortable it is, how calm and serene. Will you experience pressure, a tightening, a drawing up? Remember that your body is created to give birth gently and naturally, and at the right time and place, to allow your baby's easy and serene passage into the world, so that you can for the first time hold your beautiful baby in your arms. You realise now that it's easy to decide all these things in your new confidence; and the power that gives you, and the happiness and calmness it brings you, allow you to drift deeper into peace and calmness, confidence and wellbeing.

Now you look up with gratitude to the tree with all its green leaves with their positive thoughts and happy memories, and something wonderful happens. The leaves separate and form a beautiful green picture-frame, and the picture inside that frame is you, both of you, with your baby in your arms. You look so happy and radiant, knowing that all happened just as you had visualised it. Your baby is sleeping gently in your arms, so sweet and gentle and secure, and you are filled with love and happiness.

The picture seems to float gently down from the tree and it becomes life-size as it envelops you, and now, like a miracle, you realise that this is not a picture at all. It is real – and what seemed to be a picture of you both and your baby now really is true, and you feel overjoyed at your success. Such gentle tenderness comes over you as you look down at your baby's face and it opens its eyes wide and looks into yours. All is so perfectly as you planned it to be, and you will remember this feeling over and over again until the day when it really happens. You realise your body has been specially designed to give birth naturally, easily and comfortably, so you look forward to giving birth to your baby as the most wonderful and empowering experience, and meeting your baby happily and calmly.

So in a minute it will be time to return to everyday reality, but a different reality, as you remember all you have just experienced, and the joy it gave you, and will continue to give you, as your pregnancy progresses, as you give birth to your baby, and also after your baby is born.

As I count from five to one, gently and gradually come back to the present. **Five** Becoming aware of your body again… **Four** Gently feeling tiny movements in your fingers and toes … **Three** Your eyelids begin to feel lighter … **Two** You feel alert and calm, happy and relaxed … **One** Now gently and gradually allow your eyes to open as you quietly and gently return to the present in calm confidence.

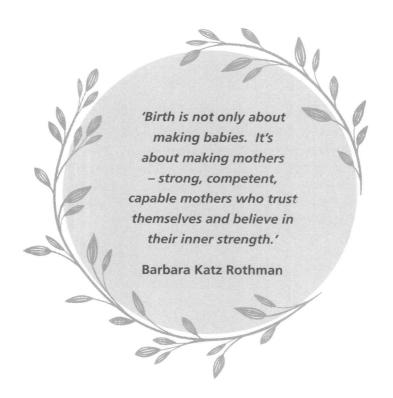

'Birth is not only about making babies. It's about making mothers – strong, competent, capable mothers who trust themselves and believe in their inner strength.'

Barbara Katz Rothman

# CHAPTER 16

# KGH Worldwide

I am delighted that we have trained people to be KGH teachers from all over the world and, now that we offer our teacher training virtually, this number is growing. This book was originally produced for couples in the UK, but since then it has been used internationally extremely effectively even though other countries may have different systems of maternity care. For example, my understanding is that gas and air is not available at home births in Sweden; the homebirth rate in the Netherlands is about 30 per cent; and the Caesarean rate in the gulf states is about 80 per cent. Many countries have an even more medicalised system of birth care than the UK, but this book is here to help you wherever you live.

Throughout this book I have referred to midwives as this is the profession that provides most of the care to pregnant women in the UK unless the protocols say an obstetrician should be called in. In many countries an obstetrician attends all, or almost all, births. In the UK a midwife is an autonomous medical professional although their autonomy is being eroded all the time and needs to be guarded. In some countries the term 'midwife' is used for someone who is effectively an obstetric nurse who does not have autonomy and carries out the instructions of an obstetrician. In some states of the USA, midwifery is actually illegal. In these states a midwife can only support you if you have a home birth and she would not be allowed to accompany you to hospital in the event of a transfer. There are very few birth centres in the USA, and most women give birth in hospital, in bed, in a recumbent or semi-recumbent position. But one of the most famous birth centres in the world, The Farm, run by Ina May Gaskin, is in Tennessee and has a much higher safety record than the American average.

Medical interventions are quickly adopted, sometimes with little research. It is very much harder to persuade hospitals to abandon the over-medicalisation of birth that has evolved, even when there is research to support this. Even the World Health Organization has issued a statement that, in the developed world, birth has become over medicalised.

Cultures and healthcare systems are different around the world. For example in some countries and cultures you may be living with your husband's family where your mother-in-law is the person in charge. She has had babies herself, and she was told what to do by her mother-in-law. Traditions of childbirth have been passed down through the generations. Without doubt your mother-in-law is looking forward to the arrival of her grandchild, but things may have been very different when she had her babies than they are now.

In your situation, your mother-in-law is part of the team. The best thing to do is to include her. Invite her to read *The Hypnobirthing Book* so she can see the logic of your approach to birth. If you are attending a virtual or face-to-face course, invite her to attend it too. If you are coming to a course that I am teaching, I would welcome her at no extra charge once you have paid the fee for you and your husband. If you are doing an online course, she can watch it too. Just as we would never advocate confrontation with your healthcare professionals and the aim is to work with your caregivers as a team, so we would always suggest that your mother-in-law is included as a valued part of your team.

Different cultures have different traditions and different terminology too. I have received abusive emails for using the word 'husband or father' rather than 'partner'. In other cultures the word 'husband' and 'father' are the only appropriate thing to say, and to use the term 'partner' would be considered insulting. I do my best, and my intention is to be welcoming to everyone. Please forgive me if I have not chosen all the right words for you.

So how do you deal with the situation wherever you are as a KGH mum? Remember that, 15 years ago, nobody in the UK knew about hypnobirthing and we hypnobirthing teachers were a small group asking ourselves, 'How do we reach the midwives?' Today, every midwife in the UK knows about hypnobirthing and many are recommending the women in their care to attend a KGH class. Now a growing number of obstetricians are attending our trainings too.

Fifteen years ago, a small group of we hypnobirthing teachers had a stand at the London Baby Show with the word 'Hypnobirthing' over it. People would see it and give us a very wide berth because we had this unknown name that implied we might do something odd to them. Three years later when we had a similar stand people were looking at the name and saying, 'My sister told me about that. Can you tell me some more?' Hypnobirthing will grow in this way in your country too, and you are part of this positive revolution.

Other countries are now in the situation that we were 15 years ago, and KGH will grow because, when a woman has a wonderful birth experience, she tells her friends. It is women that change the system, not the authorities. It may not seem that you can make much difference on your own but, over time, the more women ask questions and are well informed the quicker things will change.

I have spoken quite a lot about home birth, but in some countries, homebirth is illegal, while in other countries it is legal but very difficult to achieve in practice. I know independent midwives and KGH midwives who will travel anywhere in the world to attend a homebirth if you find it difficult to find someone to support you where you live. We can put you in touch with these amazing caregivers if you would like to consider their support when you give birth. The principles of this book are valid wherever you are. Everything we advise is evidence-based and logical. The websites quoted at the end of the book give superb information wherever you may be. Everyone in the KGH office will do their best to support you if you get in touch, and we are easily contacted on social media.

The most important thing is to ask questions, just as we suggest to women in the UK. It is even better if you have a supportive partner. You might even like to lend your copy of *The Hypnobirthing Book* to your caregivers so they understand what you are doing.

Make sure you are well informed using the acronym B.R.A.I.N.S. (see page 213 for full explanation):

**B** enefits
**R** epurcussions
**A** lternatives
**I** nformation
**N** othing
**S** mile

When making decisions remember the acronym F.A.S.T. (see page 206 for full explanation):

**F** ear. A decision made from fear tends to be a bad decision. People will play on your fear to pressurise you into agreeing to interventions that you had decided to decline.

**A** ssumptions. How often is what you call a decision actually an assumption?

**S** ocial pressure. There is a lot of this around. When it comes to birth everyone knows best.

T ime. Always take your time and never be rushed into a decision.

I know these acronyms are mentioned before in Chapter 14 but this is a reminder as, if you are having your baby in a country with a highly medicalised system, they are even more important to you.

Trust your INSTINCT as a mother. If something instinctively doesn't seem right to you, it almost certainly isn't. If something instinctively seems right to you, it almost certainly is.

And do your daily practice.

Here is the story of an Italian lady who gave birth without KGH support in a highly medicalised country and had her baby in 2 hours with only 'some discomfort'. As she said, 'If I can do it, anyone can.'

### BIRTH REPORT – ITALIAN BIRTH

*"I wanted to quickly share my experience to really say thank you. I had an amazing birth and now a wonderful baby boy. I am sure it would have been a completely different story if I haven't join your course.*

*I gave birth in Italy where unfortunately the whole process is very medicalised. Giving birth is an emergency and fear is part of it. I was offered many times during the last month of pregnancy a C-section as they could see I was terrified, and I was big time ... I was terrified since the day I realise I was pregnant as all my life I heard my mother horrible story and all my three sister had been emotionally traumatised during labour/birth all very difficult, long and painful experience.*

*As the youngest female of the family I was sure it was going to be the same. I join your course, did the homework and try to relax as much as possible. When I heard the first "movement"...can't even call them surges as they were so mild. I guess all the work I did started to pay off, my instinct took over and I knew what I had to do. I carry on doing my own things, did the laundry, went to watch my nieces swimming, I even had a beautician appointment at 8pm (and have my baby at 2.30am by the way) and just keep on walking and moving.*

*I didn't want to go into hospital as the surges were so mild and I wanted to stay at home as long as possible but my sister insisted as they were every 2/3 min. I forgot to say that I was booked to be induced the day after so again nature took over.*

*As my sister (who has 3 babies) was lovingly insisting me to go to hospital, I agree and well, I was well on my way. I had my baby 2 hours later, with a 2 hours labour which was virtually pain free and very natural, I had no pain relief and really didn't ask for it.*

*I'm sorry my English is not my first language but really wanted to pass on that if I can make it, everybody can and thank you."*

# Takeaways

❋ Medical practices and even laws are different in different countries, but KGH will still work for you.

❋ Your Mother-in-law can and should be part of your birthing team if you live with her and if she is heavily involved in your pregnancy. Invite her to join you to learn more.

❋ KGH is growing in countries all around the world. You are part of the revolution!

# CHAPTER 17

# The Onset of Labour

It is generally thought that labour starts at the baby's instigation; when the baby releases hormones into the mother's system, which triggers the mother's hormones, and after that it is a magical dance between the mother's and baby's hormones interplaying with each other.

This happens when the baby is entirely ready for the world, when his or her little heart, lungs, kidneys, liver and particularly its brain are completely ready. Of course, the baby is often viable several weeks before this, but it seems very presumptuous to think we know best, unless there is a very clear clinical reason that medical intervention is needed in an individual case. It is known that there is considerable brain development in the last few weeks of pregnancy, so, unless there is a clinical reason to the contrary, there is a strong argument to allow this development to take place in its own time. The baby also lays down a store of adipose tissue (fat) in late pregnancy to see it through birth and its transition into the world. Consider for a moment what could be the effect of pre-empting this process by bringing the baby into the world before this development has taken place.

## A show

One sign that labour can be starting is a 'show'. This is when the mucous plug – mucous and possibly slightly bloody – that seals the cervix, the neck of the womb, in pregnancy drops out because the cervix has begun to soften and open and the muscles no long hold it in. It may drop out into the toilet so you don't notice it. Having a show doesn't necessarily mean your baby will be born immediately; it could happen a week before you go into labour, but it does mean your body is beginning to prepare to give birth. Many women, however, particularly second-time mothers, could be found to be already 1cm dilated if they were examined a week before they went into labour. It doesn't mean they are in labour; it simply means the muscles are practising and beginning to soften.

## Membranes releasing

Another sign that labour is beginning is when your membranes release, or waters break. This simply means that the amniotic sac, the bag of membranes, has released the amniotic fluid around the baby. The release of fluid is generally either a great gush or a steady flow of clear fluid. Although it is usually obvious if your waters have broken, you can check if you are not sure. Simply wear a sanitary pad to absorb any fluid that may be weeping out, and a midwife will be able to tell you whether your waters have indeed broken. If you believe what you see on the movies or TV, you might think that the membranes always release at the onset of labour. The movies are drama, not real life.

Membranes can release as a first sign that labour is starting, at any time during labour, or they may still be intact when the baby is born, in which case the midwife will simply scoop the membranes off the baby's head. Any of these situations is perfectly normal. The percentage of labours starting with the release of membranes seems to be increasing, possibly because of the number of membrane sweeps that are being performed which can unintentionally (or perhaps sometimes intentionally) disturb the amniotic sac and cause the waters to break earlier. If the membranes release, it is likely that you will go into labour quite soon; most women will go into labour within 24 hours.

The membranes and the amniotic fluid around the baby have several purposes. They protect the baby from physical trauma. The fluid provides physical protection around the baby so, if you forget how big you are and bang into a doorpost, your baby will be fine because of this protection. The fluid also keeps the baby at a fairly even temperature. So if you are pregnant in Rio in the summer and the temperature is 40°C, your baby will stay comfortably cool. If you are pregnant in Alaska in the winter where it's -30°C, the fluid will keep your baby well insulated and warm.

Inhaling and exhaling the fluid also helps your baby's lungs to develop. The fluid gives space for your baby to move so that as the limbs develop, and he or she has can practise using them. This wouldn't be possible if the baby were held tightly by the powerful muscles of the uterus.

The bag of membranes also keeps the baby in an environment that is free from infection. As soon as the membranes have released, this is no longer the case, but your body does still continue to produce amniotic fluid, which will continue to be released downwards, gently flushing possible infections away from your baby.

If your membranes release as the first sign of labour you will be asked to call your midwife to let her know, and she will either visit you at home or you will be asked to go into the hospital if that is where you are planning to give birth. This is not an emergency so you can take your time. If it is the rush hour or the middle of the night you can be checked as soon as convenient.

There is one important thing to bear in mind about this. If anything is introduced into the vagina, even a sterile surgical glove, it could transfer an infection to your baby, so it makes sense to think carefully about whether you agree to a vaginal examination at this stage.

10% of women showed some signs of infection in labour if they had not gone into labour 48 hours after membrane release, but 20% of mothers showed some signs of infection after 8 vaginal examinations, which are more frequent if labour has been induced (Seaward 1997.)

For this reason, it makes sense to have no internal examinations after the waters release, as each one increases the chance that an infection such as Group B Streptococcus (GBS) may be introduced into the vagina. Even if the examination is done with sterile surgical gloves, it could transfer an infection from the vulva into the vagina.

GBS is an infection that occurs in the vulva or vagina of about 20 to 30 per cent of women. It can be transient, so if it were found to be present at 30 weeks pregnant, it might not be there at 40 weeks, and vice versa. This is why it is not routinely tested for in some countries. GBS does no harm to the mother, but in very rare cases it can cause a meningitis-type infection and brain damage or even death in a baby. 1 in 17,000 babies in the UK die from the infection (RCOG 2013:1). The greatest risk is in preterm babies, and safety is increased 10-fold after the baby reaches 37 weeks, so the longer the gestation the safer the baby. However, the vast majority of babies born to mothers after their waters have released for an extended time are absolutely fine and healthy. It should be remembered that the infection can also be carried on surfaces surrounding the baby or even on staff handling the baby so it is not necessarily the case that the infection is passed from the mother.

If your waters break and you have not gone into labour within 24 hours, it will be assumed that you will have the routine interventions according to the NICE guidelines which are induction after 48 hours and intravenous antibiotics every 4 hours during labour. This improves the protection of the baby from Group B Strep, but antibiotics carry their own risks. The problem with antibiotics is that they can greatly reduce the beneficial bacteria as well as the harmful bacteria. The immune system is largely modulated in the gut. If you damage the bacteria in the mother's gut you weaken her immune system. The antibiotics used to treat GBS are narrow spectrum and so will have less effect on the gut flora, but they will also have less effect on other potential infections such as listeria and e-coli. The administration of antibiotics may also include damage to the baby's gut flora which is the basis of the baby's immune system, and future problems such as asthma, obesity, allergy, eczema and obsessive compulsive disorder can result.

In the event that you choose to take antibiotics, it is very important for you to take good-quality probiotics afterwards to re-inoculate the gut, otherwise the gut may become colonised by any opportunistic bacteria. I am delighted to say that recently I have heard of two hospitals that do provide probiotics after the administration of antibiotics, which is an encouraging step.

Natural remedies that women have used to prevent infection are garlic, probiotics, giving birth in water, and vaginal douching. There have also been studies assessing the safety of simply waiting and allowing the baby to arrive in its own time.

As you can see, this is a complex subject and it is best to be well informed before you go into labour as many of you will have to make a choice in this situation. It is rather late to start doing research when your waters have already broken and labour is about to begin. I would strongly suggest that you read the book *Group B Strep Explained* by Sara Wickham so you understand that you do have choices and what those choices are. This book gives an unbiased assessment of the situation. If anyone tells you at this stage that there is only one safe course of action for your baby, they are not well informed and are not giving you the full picture.

In such a situation you need to ask, 'What are the risks of having an induced labour?' so you can set them against the risks of Group B Streptococcus and make an informed choice. Ask questions and ask for statistics. Then you can sensibly weigh up the risks and benefits against each other and make your decision. Make sure you feel comfortable with what you decide.

Here is an excerpt from an article in *Mothering* magazine (2003) about GBS and the effect of antibiotics, given to the mother during labour, on newborn babies:

'Some studies have shown a decrease in GBS infection in newborns whose mothers accepted intravenous (IV) antibiotics during labour, but no decrease in the incidence of death. Still other research has found that preventative use of antibiotics is not always effective. In fact, one study found no decrease in GBS infection or deaths in newborns whose mothers were given IV antibiotics during labour.

Perhaps the greatest area of concern to medical researchers, as it should be to us all, is the alarming increase in antibiotic-resistant strains of bacteria. Antibiotic-resistant bacteria can cause infections in newborns that are very difficult to treat. Many large research studies have found not only resistant strains of GBS, but also antibiotic-resistant strains of E. coli and other bacteria caused by the use of antibiotics in labouring women. Some strains of GBS have been found to be resistant to treatment by all *currently used forms of antibiotics.*

*While many studies have found that giving antibiotics during labour to women who test positive for GBS decreases the rate of GBS infection among newborns, research is beginning to show that this benefit is being outweighed by increases in other forms of infection. One study, which looked at the rates of blood infection among newborns over a period of six years, found that the use of antibiotics during labour reduced the incidence of GBS infection in newborns but increased the incidence of other forms of blood infection. The overall effect was that the incidence of newborn blood infection remained unchanged.'*

So, as you can see, there are no easy answers, and if anything is presented to you as being the only course of action that is safe for your baby, it really isn't that simple. Some mothers feel more comfortable taking antibiotics while others prefer to wait. I have heard of mothers waiting for anything up to seven days and have their baby normally and in good health. Yes, there are risks, but the risks are not all on one side. We know there are risks and benefits to both courses of action. In many cases, nature knows best, but occasionally we can be grateful for help.

This is an important subject as it is estimated that, for 10–20% of women, release of membranes is the first sign of labour. It is too late to inform yourself at the time if you are in the 1 in 5 women who find themselves in this situation. An excellent section on this included in *The AIMS Guide to Induction of Labour* by Nadia Higson, and Sara Wickham's book *Group B Strep Explained* is also a recommended source of information.

The NICE guidelines on the subject are useful:

*'Women with prelabour rupture of membranes at Term should be offered a choice of induction of labour ... or expectant management.'*

Many women seem to have been given the impression that they do not have any choice and that they have to agree to induction of labour after 24 hours.

## Surges (contractions or uterine waves)

The most usual way of going into labour is when tightenings start in your abdomen. Probably in late pregnancy the muscles of your abdomen have been tightening from time to time. Sometimes they go really hard, and then slacken off. The more you progress in pregnancy, the more often these waves of activity of the uterine muscles happen, and then one day the surges seem to come quite frequently and become more regular, and you begin to time it, and the tightening comes every half hour, then every 20 minutes, then 15 minutes, then every 10 minutes ... and then it stops, just when you thought your baby really was on its way. A couple of days later exactly the same thing happens, but this time it goes on, and it really is the beginning of your baby's arrival in the world.

Contractions can begin in a completely different way, because everyone is different. I have known mothers who were not sure if labour had started or not, then the baby arrived. Another mother went out with her husband for a meal and to the cinema at about week 39. She came home, lay down in bed, and instantly her surges started, five minutes apart and one minute long, five minutes apart and one minute long, on and on. The rhythm never varied throughout the whole of her labour, so she knew exactly when her labour started. Very efficient! But labour seldom starts like this.

More often than not you are not quite sure if your baby is

really coming, or if it isn't, or perhaps it is; perhaps we ought to call the midwife; no, it's not really worth it just yet – you are not sure if labour has started or not. If you're not sure, it's too early to call the midwife. Always wait as long as you possibly can before calling the midwife or going into hospital, because so often labour can slow down at that point.

It is possible to get an app to time surges, but I would advise against this. As soon as a machine is involved the focus switches from your body and your experience to the machine. You or your partner can time and record the surges for half an hour or an hour and then focus on your relaxations and visualisations. A couple of hours later you can repeat this.

## Takeaways

* A show is one sign of the onset of labour, but it can happen up to a week before going into labour.
* Release of membranes, or your waters breaking, is another sign that your baby is on its way and labour is likely to start within 24 hours.
* Your waters can break at any time during labour and sometimes not until your baby is born. Sometimes it's a gush, sometimes a steady flow. Real life is not like the movies.
* Internal examinations after your waters have broken can raise the risk of infections, such as Group B Strep.
* If your waters break and labour does not start within 24 hours, there are alternatives which can be equally safe as induction of labour.
* The third sign of the onset of labour is surges starting, but they can also start and stop several times in the days and weeks before giving birth.
* Resist the urge to monitor surges with an app or other device: this shifts the focus away from your own experience.

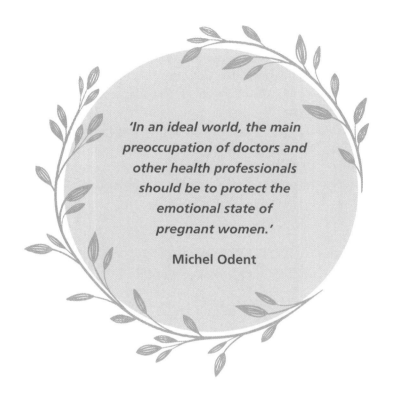

'In an ideal world, the main preoccupation of doctors and other health professionals should be to protect the emotional state of pregnant women.'

Michel Odent

# CHAPTER 18

# The Up Stage of Labour

When a baby is conceived, two things happen. It is an important and miraculous physical event, and it is an intensely personal and intimate relationship. When a baby is born, it is also an important and miraculous physical event, as well as a personal and intimate relationship. Does our system of maternity care sufficiently support the personal and intimate side of birth? Does labour progress more easily if we acknowledge this important aspect of birth?

In the up (first) stage of labour, as we saw earlier, the upper muscles of the uterus are working to draw up, which is why I call it the 'up' stage of labour which I'm delighted to see other people have subsequently adopted. At the same time, the internal muscles of the cervix release, so these muscles become thinner and are drawn back until the cervix is fully open. Now the uterine muscles have been gathered at the top of the uterus to help your baby move in a downward direction through the birth canal and out into the world. This is called the second or 'down' stage of labour.

For most people their reality of birth comes from the movies. This is not reality, it's drama. Birth is a gentle progression, and you can find some gentle hypnobirthing births on YouTube. Watch them so you can see what birth is really like.

## Early labour

In early labour, gently keep doing whatever you feel like. Continue whatever you were doing before labour began, or anything at all as long as it is gentle, or you can have a rest, and the *Confident and Positive Relaxation* script (page 220) is perfect to have read to you now. Most of the work of the scripts is done before labour, but you may enjoy having one read to you in early labour as well. You can stream one of the funny movies you have prepared to help relax the body and mind in early labour, and remember that laughter produces oxytocin. You can play the *Ultimate Birth Relaxation* audio quietly in the background because you're used to relaxing to the sound, and so is your baby. You might like to go for a gentle stroll, or rest between surges.

You need your energy for the later stages of labour. I've heard of plenty of mothers who have walked when labour appeared to be starting to try and 'get things going' and then wished they hadn't afterwards when they realised they had wasted energy and caused problems further down the line by interfering with this amazing process.

Do you remember what that Italian lady did in her birth report (page 231)? She finished doing the washing, went to watch her nieces swimming, and had a beautician's appointment. Then she had what she described as a 'virtually pain free' labour in two hours. It could be that the beautician's appointment contributed to her amazing birth story. If you know someone near you who does reflexology, massage, etc. why not give them a call, tell them you are in early labour, and that you would really appreciate an appointment (even 20 minutes would be great) if they can fit you in to help you chill out in preparation for the birth.

It's a good idea to snack, so do raid the fridge. A light snack will keep your energy up. Also sip at water to keep hydrated. It's a good idea to have a drinking straw available so you don't have to change position to have a drink. This applies particularly in later labour when you might be more comfortable on your hands and knees. If she hasn't had any water for a couple of hours, partners, just suggest quietly that it might be an idea to have a sip.

There will come a time when you may find the up breathing that you have been practising helps to relax and calm you, and helps you to produce oxytocin. The up visualisations that you learnt with this breathing ensure that mind and body are working together, so you may find it helpful to bring them to mind, or else have your birth companion gently remind you of them during surges. Or you may prefer that people don't talk to you unless you ask. The purpose of the *Ultimate Birth Relaxation* audio is to have it playing quietly in the background now which helps you subconsciously to go back into that deeply relaxed state you were in when you listened to the audio each night.

Movies portray labour as an emergency, with people rushing about and blue flashing lights on ambulances. It isn't an emergency. It is a quiet time for you to go gently further and further into yourself. There is plenty of time. Just because a woman is having a baby, it doesn't mean that she doesn't know if she is thirsty or wants a rest. In fact, her intuitive awareness of her needs and the needs of her baby are much heightened and should be treated with the greatest respect.

You are usually advised to call the midwife to come to you or to go into hospital when the surges are about three or four minutes apart, one minute long, and regular for about 30 or 40 minutes. Don't go to hospital too soon. First-time mothers tend to go into hospital far too soon. Labour often slows down as a result and they are sent home again.

It is usually the partner who makes the call and the person on the other end will say, 'Can I speak to her?' KGH mothers are usually calm and therefore the person can be confused and think she is not in established labour because she is carrying on a perfectly normal conversation rather than stopping every few minutes for heavy breathing while she has a surge. You can deal with this in different ways. It is important that you tell the person who answers the call that you are doing KGH. These days people are more used to KGHypnobirthing and they may well understand that mothers doing hypnobirthing can be in very well-established labour but still remain calm and carry on a perfectly coherent conversation.

Sometimes if you are planning a homebirth, they will say they are too busy to send a midwife so you will have to come into the unit. Note the phrase 'You will have to.' When you think about this for a minute, that is the time you particularly do not want to be in the unit because, if they are so busy, each midwife may be looking after two or three mothers. They will be extremely rushed and you will certainly not get one-to-one personalised care. If you stay at home you will get one-to-one care, because an experienced midwife is sent out just for you. This could be the time for your partner to display their protective instinct. A firm requirement if this happens has been known to work. A midwife's professional undertaking is to support you when you give birth wherever or whenever that may be.

## Place of birth

It has been said that the best environment for giving birth to a baby is the same as the best environment for conceiving a baby. The environment for conceiving a baby includes privacy, plenty of time (no rush), low lights, soft music, gentleness, stroking. The same applies to birth. Conceiving a baby is a major physical event. It is also a huge private, subtle and personal event. What is the physical aspect of conception without the personal and subtle? Birth is also an important physical event and also a private, subtle and personal event. It is important to preserve the subtle elements of birth for it to be the truly satisfying experience that it is designed to be for you and your baby.

Nobody doubts that a healthy mother and healthy baby are the most important outcomes. Surviving and thriving are two different things, and it is so important that we support thriving as well as surviving. There is every reason why mother and baby can experience both.

One-to-one care during labour from a known and trusted midwife makes a profound difference to the experience and outcome of labour. With one-to-one care a woman is less likely to have a forceps or ventouse delivery, or a Caesarean; she is more likely to have a spontaneous vaginal birth without requiring drugs; labour has been shown to be shorter; and the baby has a higher Apgar score at birth meaning that it is in a better state of health.

Sadly, in many hospitals these days you don't get this care, because the staff are too busy and there is a shortage of midwives, although they do try. One way of getting one-to-one care on the NHS is to have your baby at home, because a midwife is sent out just for you. She will probably be an experienced midwife, because she is sent out to you on her own. A second midwife will arrive to assist her in late labour, in time for the birth.

It is also true that homebirth midwives have chosen to work in this way because they are more in favour of supporting normality and want the freedom to use their professional knowledge and experience to work in this way. There is a move in the UK to establish caseloading, a system where each woman has a nominated midwife and will get to know two or three back-up midwives during her pregnancy so that, when she goes into labour, she will already know the person caring for her. This system is most likely to be set-up for homebirths.

If you decide to have your baby at home, you will have exactly the same technical support as you have in a midwife-led unit (or birth centre). You have the same pain relief available: gas and air, a tens machine and certainly a birth pool. Babies breathe spontaneously at birth (unlike what you see in the movies) but your midwife has the skills and the bag and mask to help them take their first breath in the tiny number of cases where this may be needed. The midwife will bring with her the injection to use in the rare event of haemorrhage, though this is less likely to happen at home where birth progresses without medical interventions. She can also suture if needed and carries the local anaesthetic with her.

In a labour ward or delivery suite in hospital they offer epidurals, ventouse and forceps deliveries, and Caesarean sections. But if you are reading this book it is likely that you are planning a natural birth and the place you are most likely to achieve this is your home. Some women go to a midwife-led unit or birth centre, because that is where you get the homely rooms and the birthing pools. Why do they make the rooms more like home? It is an acknowledgement that home is best because a mother feels more relaxed at home and so labour progresses more smoothly. Oxytocin, which makes labour more efficient, has been called the 'shy hormone' because you produce it when you feel unobserved and are in a situation of privacy. If you have your baby at home, you are in your own environment you have everything there that makes you feel comfortable and at ease. And you can sleep in your own bed afterwards. So you get everything that you would get in a midwife-led unit, plus the huge advantage of one-to-one care and privacy. It can be difficult to understand in advance how important that is because you do not see it in the dramatic representations of birth in the movies, but it is of paramount importance.

I have talked quite frequently about homebirth in this book, and you are very likely thinking that's not for you. Before I taught KGH I thought the same. Over the years I have had reports from many women about the birth of their babies and I can say with confidence that reading this book and doing the KGH course will make a great difference whether the baby is born in a hospital, in a birth centre, or at home. I have also become clear that the most ecstatic reports tend to come from the home births, which is why I mention it here. When I observed this, I looked at the research, and the recent research shows that homebirth is as safe, or often safer than, a hospital birth, for a normal healthy woman. There is a resource sheet which gives you information on good, evidence-based articles on this at the end of the book, and I would urge you to read this before you make your choice.

A woman often tells me, 'I would love to have my baby at home, but he (her partner) doesn't want me to.' As a partner, your role is not to tell the birthing woman what to do but to support her in her choice. Trust her instinct. Look at the evidence.

## Short triggers to take you back into your deeply relaxed state

Let's just recap on the short and effective triggers for relaxation that we have drawn out of the relaxations in this book. Realise and remember which of these work best for you and understand, through practice, how they all work differently on your body and mind and how they can be used at different stages of your pregnancy and your birthing experience. In early labour there is plenty of time for your partner to read you one of the relaxations you have practised. In established labour when the surges may be four or five minutes apart there isn't time for a full relaxation, so use the little triggers from each relaxation that can take you back into that deeply relaxed state in just a second or two because of the practice you have done.

Relaxation triggers may be:

- **Lavender:**
  Diffusing essential oil of lavender while you practise
- **Breathing:**
  Slow, gentle up breaths
- **Beautiful Pink Rose:**
  Soft and open
- **Sssoften Relaxation:**
  Your partner's voice speaking slowly and soothingly
  The word sssoften
- **Stroking Relaxation:**
  Gentle stroking of your arm, your forehead or any other part of your body you find comforting
- **Calming Touch Relaxation:**
  The feeling of a hand on your abdomen
  Someone gently raising and releasing your hand
- **Your relaxing colour**
- **Garden of Pregnancy Relaxation:**
  A beautiful posy of colourful flowers
  Three long, slow, gentle breaths with positive words
- **You Are in Control Relaxation:**
  Press together the thumb and finger
- **The Magic Carpet Relaxation:**
  Imagine any place that you would really like to be that you can drift off to on your magic carpet
- **Positive Birth Affirmations:**
  Repeat them to yourself, put them up around your home or carry them with you on cards to read

- **The 5Cs Relaxation:**
  Recall the words choice, control, confidence, calm, comfort
- **Gentle Back Stroking**

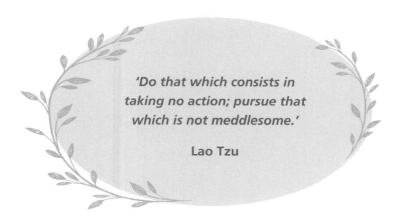

*'Do that which consists in
taking no action; pursue that
which is not meddlesome.'*

**Lao Tzu**

## Takeaways

❋ Take your time in early labour – if you rush into hospital too soon, labour may stall and you will be sent home again.

❋ You are most likely to receive one-to-one care in a home birth, where a dedicated midwife will be sent to your home.

❋ Privacy facilitates a straightforward labour. This is important – very important. It is not dramatic, and you don't see it in the movies, but privacy can make more difference than anything else..

❋ Remind yourself of your helpful short triggers, which can take you quickly into the deeply relaxed state you have practised.

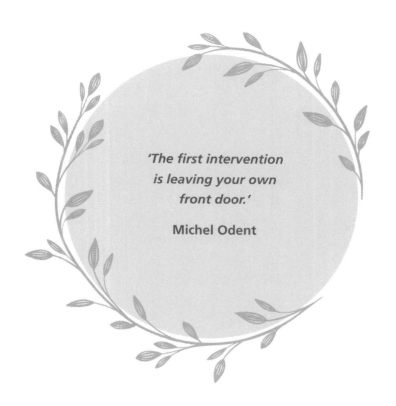

'The first intervention
is leaving your own
front door.'

Michel Odent

# CHAPTER 19

# If You Decide to go to Hospital

People often worry about transferring from home to hospital if they book a homebirth; it's one of the 'What ifs'. They have an image of blue flashing-light emergencies. There are risks at homebirths; there are risks at hospital births. The risks are different, and they are tiny, and research shows that home is safer for a normal healthy woman. For a normal, healthy woman, going to a hospital to have her baby is an intervention from the normal course of labour. It is the only time someone goes to hospital when they are not ill. You can find some suggestions for further reading on the KGH resource sheet about homebirth at kghb.org/sheets.

One of the main risks of a hospital birth is infection; you have built immunity to your home microorganisms and this is automatically passed to your baby. People go to hospital with any number of infections to which you do not have immunity.

There are also iatrogenic risks, due to the greater likelihood of medical procedures which then leads to the 'cascade of interventions'. The Birth Place Study (2011) showed that a normal healthy woman was four times as likely to end up with a Caesarean if she planned to give birth in hospital than if she planned to give birth at home. Similar results were shown for other interventions too.

Most people go to hospital for something to be done, so that is the ethos of the hospital environment and the medical profession. When you give birth you don't want 'something to be done', as your body and your baby know exactly what to do. Some women say, 'I would feel safer in hospital,' but could this just be the assumption you have been programmed with from an early age?

## Transfer

The most common reason for transfer from home to hospital is that labour is taking longer than the guidelines state (by definition not an emergency) and the second most common is that the woman requests an epidural, but these reasons seldom apply to KGH mothers. KGH labours are often quicker so the woman does not reach this cut-off time and, if she does, her well-trained KGH partner will politely enquire if the midwife is suggesting transfer because she has a concern or it is simply to comply with guidelines. If the latter, the mother can decline, and the midwife will record this in the notes to cover herself, so she has been seen to comply with the guidelines.

The second reason for transfer may be that a woman wants an epidural. It is also almost unknown for a KGH mother to transfer because she wants an epidural if she has done her practice in pregnancy. People often ask me, 'If I do KGHypnobirthing, am I allowed drugs?' The answer is, 'Yes, of course you are, but most people find they don't need them, particularly if they give birth in a pool.' It is interesting how often the word 'allow' is used in this and other contexts. Notice if you find yourself using it. It is you that does the allowing, not your caregivers.

The third reason for transfer is meconium in the amniotic fluid. Meconium is the sticky black substance that a baby passes in the first few days of life before its stools become soft and yellow from digesting milk.

The presence of meconium in the amniotic fluid means the baby has had a bowel movement before or during labour, which is an indication of a mature baby or possibly of stress. It is difficult to know which is the cause as a mother has often been subjected to a great deal of stress if she has had a longer pregnancy and the baby is obviously more mature in this situation. It is worth bearing in mind that a more mature baby may well thrive better after birth.

The guidelines these days are that, if the amniotic fluid is clear, all is well; if the amniotic fluid has a brownish tinge but is still fluid, all is well; but if there is thick, sticky meconium in the amniotic fluid, there could be a possibility of the baby inhaling the meconium, meconium inhalation syndrome, so the advice is then to transfer to hospital as a precautionary measure.

Remember that, before and during birth, your baby is receiving its oxygen through its navel and not through its lungs, and this continues for a short while after birth while it is starting to breathe normally. Remember, too, that all midwives are trained to deal with this situation and they spend a week every year making sure that their skills are up to date. A transfer to hospital would be precautionary.

If you have a homebirth you have a midwife one-to-one just for you and so, if there should be a reason for transfer, she will pick it up quickly. Most transfers are not an emergency, so you would travel by car with your partner, with your midwife following behind in her car. Your midwife has a direct line to call an ambulance if necessary, and she would call ahead to the hospital to tell them why you are transferring in so they would be ready when you arrive. She may travel in the ambulance with you or she may travel in her car, with your partner following in your car with your bags and baby car seat ready for coming home later.

If you are in a hospital, there may not be a midwife with you all the time, so it might be 15 or 20 minutes before she comes into the room and picks up if there is anything that should be done in the event of something unusual happening. She will then have to call for support and muster the team, which will take 10 or 15 minutes, so it could take as long, or possibly even longer, to get support if you are in a hospital or birth centre than if you are at home. Of course it depends where you live. If you are two hours from the nearest hospital you may make a different assessment than if the hospital is ten minutes away.

The statistics given for transfer from homebirth for first babies is roughly 40 per cent and very much less for those having a second or subsequent baby. All the teams I have asked have given a rate very much lower than 40 per cent so it puzzles me where this figure comes from. It is certain, however, that it varies from trust to trust, so find out what the figure is in your area. All the ones I have asked have had a much lower transfer rate of 10 to 25 per cent. With an experienced independent midwife the transfer rate will be very much lower. Ask your individual homebirth team what their transfer rate is. The majority of those transfers are because of 'slow progress', but this is unlikely to apply to KGH mums as it seems that our mums often give birth very much more quickly. The statistics mean that more than 60 per cent of first-time homebirths and more like 95 per cent of second or subsequent births take place normally and naturally. Any hospital would be delighted with these statistics, as interventions, even for normal healthy women, are more likely in an obstetric unit. If you transfer to hospital in labour, it is only what you would have done if you had at planned to give birth there anyway and, if that were the case, the transfer rate would be 100 per cent. Consider these facts carefully.

It is interesting to note that in 1992 a House of Commons investigation concluded that, 'On the basis of what we have heard, this Committee must draw the conclusion that the policy of encouraging all women to give birth in hospitals cannot be justified on grounds of safety,' and subsequent research has confirmed this.

Going to hospital to have your baby is an intervention from the normal course of labour.

## Travelling to hospital

If you decide to give birth in hospital, the transfer during labour can slow down or even reverse labour, so wait until you are in well-established labour before going. Many mothers feel they are in well-established labour and go to hospital, only to be told they are only 1cm dilated and sent home again. I often wonder how many of these mothers really were in established labour when they left home, but it was the unnatural experience of leaving the safety of their home, travelling in a car, and going to a strange place to be examined by strangers (however kind) that caused the whole process to reverse. We shall never know, but it is certainly something that the female of no other species would do.

One of the benefits of booking a homebirth is that the midwife will come to you to establish if you are in labour rather than you having to go to the hospital. The advantage of this is obvious. The other advantage is that, when you are in labour, you might not want to leave your home and, if you have booked a homebirth, you have left this option open to make your choice at the time. The reality when you are in labour can be very different from the assumptions you made about birth in pregnancy, so keeping your options open is very sensible.

The transfer tends to inhibit the production of oxytocin and stimulate the production of adrenaline. Leaving your home, your safe place, having strangers around, the noise of traffic, bright lights all tend to inhibit labour because they cause you to produce adrenaline and inhibit the production of oxytocin. Wear dark glasses during the transfer to block out the bright lights and listen to the *Ultimate Birth Relaxation* audio on headphones to block out the loud sounds.

Travelling on the back seat of the car with your head down in the yoga pose of the child can be more comfortable. Just do what is most comfortable. If the police stop you because you are not wearing a seat belt I think they may well let you go on when they discover why!

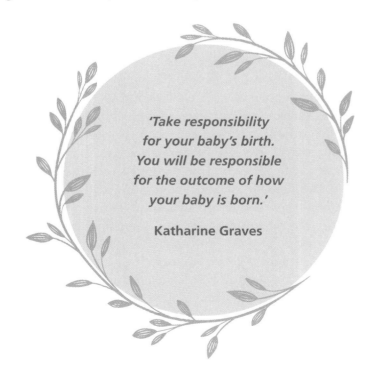

'Take responsibility
for your baby's birth.
You will be responsible
for the outcome of how
your baby is born.'

**Katharine Graves**

## Hospitals

Keep your dark glasses on when you arrive at hospital as the blue LED lights also inhibit oxytocin. Continue to listen to your audio on headphones to block out the hospital sounds. Do everything possible to take your bubble of positivity with you. You will have the process of triage (checking in), which can take some time if they are busy. Some hospitals have a triage room where you wait until a midwife is free to see you, and others do triage in the room where you will give birth. You may have the impression from your antenatal hospital tour that you arrive at the hospital and are instantly ushered into your lovely room. This depends if there is a midwife available and how busy they are. You may find you are waiting for quite some time. So practise your up breathing and do your visualisations, as you do in KGHypnobirthing throughout the up (first) stage of labour. Your partner can stroke your arm and gently remind you of the triggers from the relaxations you practised.

Check beforehand the time when the shift changes in the hospital. At that time you may be kept waiting even longer in triage while midwives look at notes and hand over cases to their replacements. In many hospitals this is at 8am and 8pm.

People may come in and out of your room from time to time, and you will be able to hear doors banging and voices in the corridor, as well as the woman in the room next door.

If you are going to an obstetric unit or a birth centre to have your baby, take one or two things with you to make it as much like home as possible. You might take a pillow, or some clothing from your partner or older child. Smell is a very basic primal sense, and it can make a big difference to how you settle into a new environment. A photo from your bedside table can also be nice. Old, baggy T-shirts can be comfortable to wear rather than a hospital gown.

Make sure you remember the beautiful picture of a full-blown pink rose that we spoke about earlier, and also something, a scarf, piece of paper, etc., of the colour that has become your relaxing colour in the *Calming Touch* relaxation. Take your KGHypnobirthing folder too.

## Takeaways

✳ Consider the reasons for possible (unlikely) transfer to hospital from a homebirth so you can make an informed choice about place of birth.

✳ If you decide to give birth in hospital, make the journey as calm as you can. Wear dark glasses to filter out bright lights, listen to your relaxing audio on headphones to block out loud or harsh noises, and keep your glasses and headphones on until you are in your room.

✳ Booking a homebirth keeps your options open so you can make your choice at the time.

✳ Triage can take a while when arriving at hospital, especially if you arrive close to the shift change. Your partner can stroke your arm while you listen to your audio to help you remain calm and comfortable.

✳ It's a good idea to bring some things to help you to settle in and to make your hospital room as much like home as possible. Clothes and photographs are easy to pack and effective, and your own pillow can make a huge difference. Your picture of a pink rose. Something to remind you of your relaxing colour. Your KGHypnobirthing folder.

# CHAPTER 20

# Choices in Labour

Plan your labour logically and carefully. The knowledge you have from this book and the KGH class is invaluable to help you. Of course circumstances may change, but how you set up the experience in advance is of great importance.

## Birthing pools

Many mothers have found that giving birth in water is much more comfortable. I have heard it said that the effect of a birthing pool is as good as an injection of an opioid – and with none of the harmful effects. The benefits are you are less likely to tear, labour is often quicker, the water supports your weight, you are likely to be in a good position to give birth, kneeling and leaning on the edge of the pool, and it is more comfortable. Also, from the emotional and psychological aspect (and you now know how important this is) the pool has become your safe place, your nest.

If you are having your baby at home most people buy an inflatable pool although you can sometimes borrow one or hire one for a nominal fee from your local homebirth group, doula, or independent midwife. If the pool has been used before, you need to buy a new sterile liner. Pools come in two sizes, and the smaller size will be big enough. You might be able to buy a used pool on the Internet, in which case you just need to buy a new, sterile liner for it, and you can resell the pool afterwards, or donate it to your local homebirth group or independent midwife, who will make good use of it for other mothers. Many people keep it for use as a paddling pool later.

Have a practice run setting up the pool before your baby is born, to ensure everything is there and working well, and that you know how to inflate it. You want to be sure, too, that the tap fitting works on your taps. Pools come with a pump and a hose so you don't have to take ages filling them with bowls of water, and you should check that these work too. You need to partially fill the pool to work out how long it will take to fill the whole pool. It takes a long time to inflate and fill a birth pool. You can inflate it in advance of labour or as soon as labour starts but you cannot fill it in advance because of the possibility of infection.

I believe that, by now, every midwife-led unit in the UK has a birthing pool, and many obstetric units are beginning to install them too, but the question is whether the will to use the pool is there in a more medicalised environment. Mothers who need extra support in labour will benefit from the extra comfort of labouring in a birthing pool. It is gloriously relaxing.

You are usually told not to get into the pool until you are 5cm dilated. It is another occasion when the phrase 'You are not allowed' is often used; a phrase which should set off alarm bells in your head. The reason given for this advice is that you might relax so much that labour slows down. In established labour the comfort of the warm water allows any tension you are holding in your body to drop away and labour progresses more quickly. If labour did slow down because you were in the pool, I am sure you would have the intelligence to get out if that was suggested to you. Once you have decided you would like to get into the pool it is not an irrevocable decision. You can easily get out again if you want to move into a different position or simply have a rest. It's your choice.

The funny thing is that mothers who ring the hospital too early in labour are often told to go and have a nice, warm bath and relax. As soon as they get into hospital in established labour, they are told they are not allowed to get into the warm, comfortable birthing pool because it slows labour down. An interesting anomaly.

Resources in midwifery and obstetric units are often stretched. With a limited number of pools and midwifery time, it may be that, if there is a large number of women in early labour, the unit, quite reasonably – in an effort to do their best for everyone and use their resources to best advantage – will want to wait to see which mother progresses first and is therefore given access to the birthing pool as, once she is in the pool, a midwife will be with her all the time, which should be the case anyway but the reality is sometimes different because of stretched resources.

If there is no pool available, it can be comfortable to kneel in the shower. You are in a good position for maximum pelvic capacity and working with gravity, and the water cascading on your back is like a gentle massage.

## Vaginal examinations

Internal examinations are routinely offered when you first get to hospital to see how far dilated your cervix is, to check if you are 5cm dilated before you are 'allowed' to get into a birthing pool, and to see if you are fully dilated – that your cervix is about 10cm dilated – before you are 'allowed' to push. They are also offered routinely about every four hours. A woman is usually required to be flat on her back for a vaginal examination, the most uncomfortable, and least efficient, position in labour.

It is very important to remember that this, and any other intervention is 'offered'. It is entirely your choice whether to accept it. Experienced midwives, and independent midwives, will have the confidence to support you in labour safely, gently and extremely well without doing any vaginal examinations. In many cases, most cases indeed, you are absolutely fine without them. No woman likes to have a vaginal examination, they are uncomfortable and slightly embarrassing, and labour can often tend to slow down or reverse as a result.

The more experienced the midwife, the less she will rely on them. A vaginal examination simply tells her how far dilated you are at that moment. It does not tell her how, or how fast, labour will progress. There may be a particular medical circumstance where the information gained is necessary to make a clinical assessment. If this was explained to you, I am sure you would agree to an examination but the need for this is rare. Just because something is usually done, it doesn't necessarily mean that it is in your best interests. There are plenty of routine procedures done in pregnancy, labour and birth that are not evidence-based.

A mother I spoke to recently had been having mild surges (pre-labour) for two days, and then progressed from 2cm dilated to fully dilated in 10 minutes. It is equally possible that a woman could reach 7cm dilation in a couple of hours, and then everything slows down for a while. Another mother told me recently how she had two babies without a single vaginal examination at any time – two very quick and straightforward births. I wonder if the two facts could be connected?

One NHS trust's guidelines on vaginal examinations say:
▓ The woman is seen as central to decision-making about timing and frequency of vaginal examinations.
▓ Staff should ensure they are able to justify each examination.
▓ Vaginal examinations must be considered within the context of the woman's individual experience of labour and offered four hourly.

- Examinations should be carried out with sensitivity and in privacy.
- Verbal consent should be obtained and recorded in the woman's handheld healthcare records.
- The woman's right to decline examination should be respected and recorded.

The guidelines also say that vaginal examinations should be 'offered', not that they should be done, nor that you have to agree to them. If you prefer not to have a vaginal examination make sure the midwife at your next antenatal visit records it in your notes. It is also wise to write to your hospital's head of midwifery, or the appropriate consultant midwife, telling her of your decision, and asking her to make sure this is in your notes. Have a copy of the letter with you when you go into labour just to be sure this has happened. When you choose care that is less usual, it helps your midwife if she can see that the head of midwifery or other senior midwife has already been informed.

If you have your baby at home, you will probably already know the homebirth midwife, and she may be more relaxed about supporting you without doing a vaginal examination. If you decide to go to a hospital or birth centre, you will almost certainly meet a midwife you don't know and, even if you have decided to decline vaginal examinations, it may be less stressful for you to agree to one in triage so that you are admitted without too much fuss, rather than being sent home again because, as a KGH mum, you don't appear to be in labour.

I was at a hearing at the Nursing and Midwifery Council (NMC) when it was agreed by the panel that it is safe and professional to support a woman in labour without doing vaginal examinations.

## Rapport with your midwife

Another thing I would like to talk about is communication with your midwife. Midwives are kind and caring people, they are also generally extremely busy. If you don't tell them you are doing KGHypnobirthing, how are they to know? They want to support you. They wouldn't be in the profession if they didn't. The hours are demanding, and the pay is not that amazing, but it's the only job where you are present daily at a miracle.

So, I would suggest you write a note to give to the midwife who will be supporting you when you give birth. It is designed to be helpful to her. You've probably done a longer birth plan as well, but that might be tucked away in your notes and there may not be a lot of time for the staff to study it closely if the unit is busy. So, write a very short note, preferably in your own handwriting and your own words. Take several copies with you in case there is a shift change, so your partner can give a copy to anyone who comes into the room, and then everyone knows what you are doing. I would suggest it says something like this:

*We have been practising KGHypnobirthing and our focus is on a calm and natural birth. We would very much appreciate your support in this by helping us to create a calm and quiet environment at all times, both physically, mentally and emotionally, with no routine interventions and no routine vaginal examinations without fully informed consent and unless absolutely necessary.*

*We would particularly request that no coaching is given during the second stage of labour and that all conversation is kept to the absolute minimum.*

*If you have any questions, please ask .................... (insert the name of your birth partner) in the first instance, and not me.*

*Thank you so much for your help.*

*Signature*

Let's go through it:

**'We have been practising hypnobirthing and our focus is on a calm and natural birth.'**
Now the midwife knows what you are doing. Almost every woman in pregnancy will say, 'I want a natural birth; I don't like drugs', but when in labour many women ask for an epidural. Midwives have seen this time and time again. The difference between this and you as a KGH mother is that you have done something to achieve a natural birth and you are very likely to get it. More and more midwives are now beginning to have experience of KGH, and they know very well that if you have read this book and done the course, you are very likely to achieve what you want – a natural birth for you and your baby. More midwives also now understand the difference between KGH and other methods which is important. Tell her what you have been doing and she will be in a better position to support you.

**'We would very much appreciate your support in this.'**
Your midwife wants to support you, so ask for her help – so that everybody is working together.

**'... By helping us to create a calm and quiet environment at all times, both physically, mentally and emotionally.'**
People may understand about quiet rooms, soft music and low lights, but mental and emotional quietness are even more important, and unguarded words can create enormous stress. So it is a good idea to remind your midwife of the importance of this right at the beginning. It is also very helpful if your birthing partner knows about KGH, though many women

use what they learn here extremely effectively without such support. It is helpful if your birthing partner attends the course with you or at least reads *The Hypnobirthing Book*. They may well come unwillingly but leave an enthusiastic and staunch supporter of what you are doing.

### 'No routine interventions and no routine vaginal examinations without our fully informed consent unless absolutely necessary.'

I would like to reiterate that I am always talking about a normal, natural situation, and that I am not medically qualified. I am certainly not suggesting you disregard medical advice. However, as we have seen in earlier chapters, many things are done absolutely routinely and mothers say afterwards, 'If I had known I would never have agreed.' If you start from the premise that you are not going to have anything done unless it is fully explained to you and there is a particular clinical need, rather than from the assumption that you will have all the routine procedures, it can make for a gentler and more natural labour and birth.

Please note the above phrase does not say you have declined all interventions. It simply says that the starting point is that nothing will be done, but if a particular course of action is fully explained to you, then you will consider whether to give your consent. The law says that no intervention may be done without informed consent, and remember that every procedure is an intervention, however apparently benign. Information does not mean someone telling you why they think it is a good idea. It means that all the risks and benefits of the proposed procedure, plus all the risks and benefits of an alternative course of action (remember that everything has benefits and everything has risks), or of doing nothing, are fully explained to you, together with research evidence and the statistical likelihood of each.

*'We would particularly request that no coaching is given during the second stage of labour and that all conversation is kept to the absolute minimum.'*
Why is it that, for the most part, it is assumed that a mother knows how to grow and birth her baby, until it comes to the point when she is ready to ease her baby down the birth canal, and then she needs to be coached? This is completely unnecessary for a KGH mother, and even distracting, and therefore it can be harmful. Talking now disturbs the neocortex, the thinking part of the brain, stimulating the production of adrenalin which inhibits the production of oxytocin, and tending to lead to a longer and more uncomfortable birth. After the baby is born, too, it is the most special time, and conversation from the midwife is superfluous and intrusive. We will have a look at this very special time later on.

*'If you have any questions, please ask ...........* (insert the name of your birth companion) *in the first instance, and not me.'*
This little message has to come from you, the mother, because legally you are the patient and therefore instructions can only be taken from you. Of course, the midwife will also look to your partner to tell her what you want so as not to disturb you, but this phrase gives her specific authority to do that. If something is put in writing, it should be in terms that are helpful to her. Adding this message doesn't mean that decisions are taken by your partner for you. It simply means that any run-of-the-mill questions can pass you by. When you start answering questions, the thinking part of your brain clicks into gear and, as you have seen, it is activity in that part of the brain that transfers you from the confident state into the fear response. So the fewer

questions and the less that you are bothered, the better.

I remember a mother who did KGH, and who told me that she was in a birthing pool at home when her baby's heartbeat began to slow just a little. This is something that you take seriously which is why your midwife checks it regularly. The midwife said to the father in the kitchen, 'I think we should transfer to hospital.' The father talked it through with the midwife. He asked if it was an emergency or if it would be safe to have a little more time to see how things developed – a perfectly sensible question. The midwife said the change in heartbeat was only slight, and she was happy to monitor the situation carefully, and if the heartbeat was still slow in half an hour, they really should transfer.

In half an hour, and the heartbeat was back to normal. The midwife had the conversation with the husband first but of course in the event of a transfer, it would have been the mother's decision.

If somebody had told the mother in labour that there was concern because her baby's heartbeat was slowing, what would have happened? She would have gone into the fear response which inhibits the production of oxytocin, the whole labour would very likely have slowed down or stopped, and almost certainly it would have been more uncomfortable and possibly longer, and generally harder for her and for the baby. But because the conversation took place in the kitchen, the mother never knew about it until after her baby was born; an example of a professional midwife and a protective birth companion.

### 'Thank you so much for your help.'
The note finishes with your thanks. This is only courteous, because we can be extremely grateful to the midwife who is with us. She certainly deserves your thanks.

## Positions and relaxation in the up stage

This is a very important section. The two most important things when it comes to giving birth are position and relaxation. For a normal healthy woman, size of baby and length of pregnancy are of little significance by comparison.

You may find that being upright and leaning slightly forwards is the most comfortable. That might be sitting on a birth ball, leaning on a bed, kneeling in a birthing pool, or standing with your arms around your partner's neck. You may find that you feel like going for a gentle stroll, not going for a walk to 'try to make the baby come' or walking up and down stairs to 'try to get things going'. Either of these simply dissipate energy that you will need later on. You may feel like lying down and having a rest for a while. You will know what is right for you, and no-one needs to tell you.

Something that is very comforting is the stroking of your arm, as in the *Stroking Relaxation*, where your partner strokes your hand and arm. Because you have practised it in pregnancy with a deep relaxation exercise, stroking brings a much greater depth of relaxation than it would on its own. And because your partner spoke to you quietly and softly while you were relaxing, then their voice itself is what in hypnotherapy terms is called an 'anchor' for relaxation, and will help when you are having your baby.

The word 'sssoften', the hand dropping, and your relaxing colour are also tools to use now. All these things are helpful.

## Gentle back stroking

Another form of stroking that is relaxing and soothing is stroking on the back. A good way to practice this is kneeling on the sofa with your head resting on cushions on the back of the sofa, or in a similar position, and your partner stands behind you. Partners, the stroking is done very, very gently with the back of the hands – so gently it is almost as if your fingers are floating off the surface of the skin. It is a more gentle touch with the back of the hands than with the front. As lightly as you can, start on the coccyx, at the bottom of the spine, and slowly and gently move your hands straight up the centre of the back, all the way up the spine, and when you get to the top of the back, stroke outwards across the shoulders and then come down both sides of the back. Repeat this for as long as she wants. You may find she wants it for a long time because it feels so soothing when you are giving birth.

If you can't reach her back, you can do the stroking on the thighs or the abdomen instead – anywhere. But it feels particularly effective on the back for several reasons.

Obviously, you are doing nothing like a normal massage which is pummelling muscles, but what you are doing is very, very gently soothing the nerve endings under the skin. Gentle stroking helps to produce endorphins – nature's pain relief. When you go up the back, you are soothing the whole of the central nervous system. You are also working in conjunction with the meridian system that acupuncture uses, helping to balance the meridians and the energy of the body.

So in one very simple movement you are working at four different levels: soothing the central nervous system, stimulating the comfort hormones, endorphins, giving her a mini acupressure treatment and, maybe best of all, it just feels so good.

Back stroking feels lovely and is so simple; a couple of passes up the back have such a profound effect. It is a calming thing to do for each other when you come home from work each day. All the stresses of the day just fall away. In fact, it would be good if every class of schoolchildren did it first thing in the morning – then schools would be much happier places.

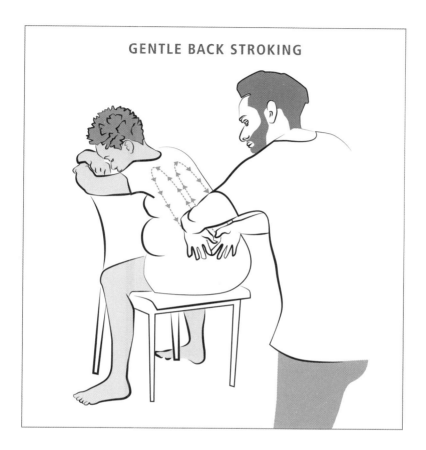

GENTLE BACK STROKING

## Natural remedies for use in labour

This section is included to give you a few simple pointers if you are interested. It may be that you are not interested, in which case leave it out. It may be that you already know a great deal more than this basic information.

Some people like to use essential oils in labour, and the one that is best known for helping you to relax is lavender. You can put a few drops in an essential oil diffuser and the calming aroma disperses into the atmosphere. If you are in hospital you would need to get an electrical diffuser as they won't allow naked flames which are a fire risk. Some hospitals offer essential oils anyway so you wouldn't have to take your own. Alternatively, you can buy essential oils in a spray to spray around the room. Some hospitals, however, don't allow the use of essential oils in the atmosphere in case the next woman in that room doesn't like the aroma; in that case, put a couple of drops on a tissue or handkerchief and hold it to your nose.

Flower remedies are also calming. Many people know of Rescue Remedy. Many therapists would recommend the Five Flower Remedy – the equivalent which is more authentically made according to the instructions of Dr Edward Bach – that you can buy online from Healing Herbs. Put just a few drops in your water container and once that's done you don't have to think about it again. You can also spray flower remedies around the room. They are very soothing.

You may find essential oils and flower remedies supportive in labour, but they can be equally helpful at other times. If you have had a stressful antenatal visit, or you have to decide whether to agree to an induction or felt pressurised in any way, or if all your friends have just called you in one morning to see if your baby has arrived yet, these remedies can help you to remain calm and composed. If your baby has been awake all night and you wonder if you are doing the right thing as a new mother, the remedies can be calming for you and for your baby.

You can also use arnica 200 in labour. Arnica is probably the best-known homoeopathic remedy and is generally used for bruising, but it can be used to support any tissue that has been under stress. However gentle your labour, your body will have been under unusual stress, and arnica can help it return to normal. You can get it from a homoeopathic pharmacy, any good health food shop, or online. Allow one pill to dissolve under your tongue from time to time during labour, one when your baby is born, and continue for a couple of days after the birth.

Always take qualified advice before using any remedies and discuss with your healthcare professionals.

## Follow your intuition

Your intuition is important and should be respected.

It is also important in early labour to put yourself in the right frame of mind. I'll tell you about one of 'my' hypnobirthing mothers. Shortly before her baby was due, she felt that she just wanted to be with her husband, who was working that day in the garden of a big house in the country. So she went and sat in the garden. There was a stream running through the garden and it was a sunny day in early summer. She could have said to herself that, though she would love to be with him, she really ought to do some work or get the baby's room ready, or do some shopping before the baby arrived. But she went with her intuition. She sat beside the stream in this garden, reading, and from time to time a fish would rise and she would watch the ripples flowing out and out until the water was smooth again. Her favourite flower was a peony, and the peonies in the garden were just coming open into full bloom, and as she and her husband went home, they picked one. She went into labour that night.

She had effectively the perfect KGH home waterbirth of three hours, with no need for drugs. But she had done everything right. She had rested. She had the soft and open visualisations fresh in her mind of the flower opening and the ripples flowing out in the stream, and she had done her practice during pregnancy. She had set herself up for the best possible birth experience, and that is what happened. This is what I mean by a mother's intuition. Do what your intuition tells you at all times. It is very important. You are the expert.

## A hypnobirthing report and the effect of being observed in labour

I would like now to share with you the story of one couple's experience of KGH. Their report is interesting on the subject of labour slowing down when you are observed. There are many other examples of how they used what they had learnt in KGH when the baby was actually on its way:

*Diana's Birth*

*I just wanted to tell you what a wonderful experience we found KGHypnobirthing to be. I've made jokes about standing on street corners wearing a sandwich board extolling the virtues of hypnobirthing, but it's not far from the truth.*

*We had our baby girl at home in our little flat with a birthing pool, which took up pretty much all of our sitting room. I spent the days before her birth preparing our home so it felt really beautiful, filled with flowers and calmness. Our telly and sofas were pushed to the side and the sitting room was filled with my favourite things and pictures. I even got round to making a cake for the midwife. [Always look after your midwife!]*

*At about seven o'clock on Friday evening (our baby was due on the Monday) I started feeling surges that were more frequent than the practice surges I had felt all week. We went to bed, but I knew that our baby was on its way.*

*At around 2am I woke up because the surges were getting stronger, and Thomas went to inflate the birthing pool. We had had a trial run a week earlier, which was really*

*helpful. We started timing the surges at around 3am, and
at 5am the midwife came over to check on my progress.
At this point I was using our bed for support, leaning over
lots of pillows with a hot water bottle against my tummy.
The midwife was lovely, supportive of our hypnobirth and
impressed by how well we were doing by ourselves. She
gave me an examination, the only one I had, and I think she
said I was 3cm dilated.*

*It was interesting for me to see that, even though I
was at home in an environment I felt so comfortable in,
with my husband by my side and everything going well, as
soon as the midwife arrived my surges slowed right down.
I was gently telling myself to stay calm and focused in my
own bubble of concentration, but the midwife's presence
had a notable impact on me. I could really feel the surges
becoming less strong and less frequent, rewinding to how
they had felt an hour earlier. Thomas spoke to the midwife
about this and we decided we would much rather continue
with my labour alone, so we could concentrate on getting
back into the bubble I needed to be in. The midwife was
happy with my progress, and happy to leave us alone
until we felt we needed more help. This was brilliant and
made all the difference for us. After she left we kissed and
cuddled, and after a while my surges returned to their
previous strength and frequency.*

*At about this point I moved to our tiny loo, where I
spent several hours. I had been getting frustrated about
how often I needed to pee, so it just seemed easier to
stay where I was rather than rushing to the loo every
20 minutes or so. Not glamorous but very comfortable.*
[This is the mother's rational explanation for this, but note
that her instinct is telling her to go to a small, safe place,
which any female will naturally do ready to have her baby.]

*I found the upward breathing very helpful at this point and found myself doing some rather strange tonal singing, which helped to relieve the build-up of energy. I think this was a really efficient part of labour and Thomas was amazingly helpful and was very supportive with my visualisations and breathing.*

*At 9am our new midwife arrived. The new midwife looking after me was wonderful. She popped her head around the loo door, introduced herself and then slipped away again. She was so respectful of our wishes and incredibly supportive of our hypnobirthing. To have her there was brilliant.*

*I got into the birthing pool and things progressed quickly. Thomas was brilliant, I really couldn't have done it without him. My surges were very powerful by now, but I can remember saying to him that I was enjoying it; sort of extraordinary, but the reality that we were about to meet our baby was starting to hit me, and it was very exciting.*

*The second phase of labour was fairly full-on but over pretty quickly,* [she said afterwards that it was when the midwife started to talk that it became more painful, and next time she would ask the midwife to be silent] *about half an hour, and Thomas and the midwife were again brilliant in supporting me through it.*

*At 1.45am our daughter was born. My husband caught her in the pool and we put her on my chest straightaway. The feeling of elation and surprise was unlike anything either of us could have imagined or could possibly describe. Just 'Wow!' Lots of tears of delight. We waited for the cord to stop pulsing before cutting it, and delivered the placenta naturally.*

*The midwife continued to be wonderful, looking after us and helping Thomas clear up the flat, which really didn't take long. It definitely wasn't the messy event I think I had been fearing – I'm a bit of a tidiness freak.*

*It was magic to be able to climb into bed a few hours after the birth of our beautiful baby and be in our own calm and beautiful home. I do use the word 'wonderful' to describe the birth of our beautiful baby, and I know there are so few women lucky enough to do that. I believe so strongly in the power of positive thought and the strength of KGH. We put in a lot of practice and it really paid off.*

*Thank you, Katharine, for teaching us. The gift of helping to give us a wonderful birth is something we really treasure.*

It brings tears to my eyes, every time I read that birth report. The couple here managed better on their own in the early stage of labour, and it is a classic example of the effect of being observed, even in the safety of their own home.

Notice that the mother says, 'we kissed and cuddled, and quite quickly my surges returned to their previous length and frequency.' Sometimes I think that when a woman is in labour, particularly in hospital in a strange environment, a father almost feels as though he is not allowed to touch her. A kiss and a cuddle are wonderful. Nobody can tense their lips while having a loving kiss and, if your lips are relaxed, so is the rest of your body. Relaxing the area of the jaw especially relates to the area of the pelvis, so it is a wonderful way of helping a mother to relax while she is giving birth.

# Transition

Then you get to the stage which is sometimes called transition. With KGH you may not notice it at all. Transition is the stage where your hormones are changing and for a short time your body may not be quite sure whether it is drawing up or bearing down, and so there may be a feeling of confusion. Occasionally I hear this stage mentioned by a KGH mother, but most frequently I don't. If you are relaxed and calm, the body can just move easily from the up stage into the down stage.

## Takeaways

* Giving birth in water has many benefits. Most people get an inflatable birth pool.
* Birth pools can sometimes be hired or bought second hand. You will just need a new liner.
* Vaginal examinations are offered and you don't have to have them. Remember that interventions and examinations are your choice.
* It's important to build a rapport with your midwife. A good midwife is supportive, but not intrusive and listens to your wishes. Make sure all your caregivers know that you are doing KGHypnobirthing.
* Find your most comfortable position for labour. Position is important.
* Back stroking is gloriously relaxing.
* Natural remedies can be helpful.
* Trust your intuition when you are giving birth. Your body will tell you what it needs and where it wants to be.
* Just being observed can have a negative effect on the progress of labour.

# CHAPTER 21

# The Down Stage of Labour, and Your Baby's Birth

When your cervix is fully dilated, your body is ready to release your baby out into the world, but you may not feel this instinct straight away. Trust your instinct. Some people call this pause the 'rest and be thankful' stage, when your body is simply taking a rest before the physical work of easing the baby on its journey through the birth canal.

There is no rush. The process of birth will start up again in its own time. Sometimes a midwife may tell you to start pushing before your body is ready. If you do this, it will only exhaust you and be inefficient. Partners, politely make sure she is given the space to take her time and follow the lead of her body and her baby.

Relaxation and position are the most important things at this stage.

## Down breathing

Because the emphasis is downwards in this second stage and the baby is moving down the birth canal, I call it the 'down' stage of labour. For the first stage of labour you use the up breathing and images, to remain calm and relaxed as the uterine muscles draw up during a surge. As you begin the down stage of labour, you start to use the down breathing as the muscles have gathered at the top of the uterus ready to ease your baby downwards and out into the world. It is a quick breath in through the nose, and a longer breath out through the nose – focusing, not forcing, downwards towards the pelvic floor. It is a much more focused way of breathing, equally relaxed as the 'up' breathing but much more focused, almost as if your breath is following your baby down. Remember as you breathe that you are not *forcing* downwards, but *focusing* downwards. Your partner can help you to remember the visualisations that go with this breathing, gently bringing to mind images that are down, soft and open. Here they are:

■ **Blossom Falling** Just imagine the blossom drifting gently down from a tree – pink, white – and forming a beautiful carpet on the ground.

■ **Autumn Leaves** If your baby is likely to be born in the autumn, you might like to bring to mind the image of autumn leaves – yellow, gold, red, brown – gently drifting downwards.

■ **Snowflakes** For a winter baby, the image of snowflakes gently dancing downwards is utterly captivating and so relaxing.

■ **Mountain Stream** Imagine sitting beside a delightful little mountain stream with the sunlight shining on the drops of water as it trickles downwards in a waterfall. (If you are in a country where there are no mountain streams, you might like to visualise a fountain instead).

For the soft and open images:

■ **Rose** (or other flower) Soft, open, smooth, velvety, utterly entrancing.

■ **Ripples** As a pebble drops into a pond, the ripples go out wide, open, smooth, fluid.

Add this breathing to your practice from about Week 36. You can also practise it when you are on the toilet, as the competition for space in your pelvis as your baby's head engages ready for birth may make you a little constipated towards the end of your pregnancy. You can prove to yourself that this breathing works before your baby is born, and it is a useful life skill!

## Pushing? – or not

The question that so many mothers ask is, 'How will I know when to push?' The simple answer is, 'You will', but that's not a very helpful thing to say. The question itself shows that people think birth is something you have to 'do' rather than a natural event that happens when it is ready. You might say, 'How do you know when you need to go to the toilet?' First you think you might, then you know that you do, then you couldn't stop it if you tried. It is similar with giving birth to a baby. Nobody needs to tell you how or when, and even some of the same muscles are used. Nobody needs to stand beside you when you're on the toilet telling you when to push – and if you try to push when your body isn't ready, nothing happens.

Another way of bringing some reality to bear on the situation is to ask, 'How do you know when to sneeze?', 'How do you know when to yawn?', 'How do you know when to blink?' These are all natural reflexes that happen automatically when your body needs to do them. Birth is the same. The only difference is that you may not have done it before, so your brain is wanting to be involved in the process in a way that doesn't actually happen at the other times.

I particularly remember a mother for whom this was a very big issue. But after the birth she told me, 'It was just obvious from one surge to the next. My primal instincts took over, and I just pushed.'

The interesting thing about this birth was that I also heard from the midwife who attended her. It was a homebirth and she was a very senior midwife, because it is often an experienced midwife who attends homebirths. Midwives who want more freedom to give woman-centred care and be less subjected to rigid controls and protocols will often choose to work in the community doing homebirths. They often get to know the women for whom they are caring better and will give them more time at prenatal visits. It was this midwife's first experience of attending a KGH birth.

My phone rang and there was a woman's voice I didn't know on the other end of the line saying something like, 'It was amazing. Just wonderful. I've never seen anything like it. It was amazing.' I thought, 'Who are you, and what on earth are you talking about?' I began to genuinely think it was a new form of telephone sales.

Finally she said, 'I was with one of your mothers last night. It was just amazing. I've never seen anything like it. I got to the house and it was quite late at night. Usually when I arrive at the house and it's a first baby, there's often a certain amount of worry and fuss going on and I have to calm them down. When I went in it was completely calm, there was soft music playing, candles burning. They were doing whatever they had been taught to do. I have no idea what it was, but they seemed entirely calm and in control, so I just sat quietly at the side and didn't interfere.' Now this was a good midwife. A really, really good midwife does very little and says even less, but knows when she is needed. She told me, 'They were doing really well, and then when it came time for the baby to be born, it just seemed to slip out. It was so easy. I've never seen anything like it.'

The mother's experience was, 'My primal instincts took over and I just pushed,' and the midwife's was, 'It was so easy. I've never seen anything like it,' and that was a very experienced midwife. Any midwife attending her first KGH birth will often make a similar comment. Plainly, the mother had been doing her focused down breathing, she had worked with her body, and everything she had learnt had worked efficiently and well.

The old-fashioned way of coached pushing as a mother gave birth used to be that somebody stood beside her and more or less shouted at her, not from any ill-will, but simply because the further a woman goes into labour the more she goes into herself, so you have to speak firmly and loudly to get through to her. It is almost as if the rest of the world doesn't exist for her. The person would put a hand on the abdomen and say, 'Now take a deep breath, put your chin on your chest, and push while I count to ten. PUSH. One, two, three, four …' This simply deprives you and therefore your baby of oxygen, and is exhausting and ineffective. Sadly this still sometimes happens.

If your midwife starts doing that – partners, stop her, politely but firmly. It is actively unhelpful. The down breathing that we have done works very well. It works on its own. This can sometimes be difficult for your midwife, who is an experienced and knowledgeable birth professional, because she can't see anything happening and she is aware the protocols dictate that there is a suggested time limit for your baby to be born once you are fully dilated, and she wants to save you from further interventions. This is an occasion for another polite explanation from your birth partner that we know the down breathing works well, as it has in thousands of cases. We also know that it can be difficult for a midwife if she hasn't seen it before, but suggest you let the mother continue with her breathing quietly and without interruption for half an hour and then re-assess the situation. Remember that KGH births are very often quicker than usual, and progress will probably be apparent within this time. To push with forced pushing of your shoulders, holding your breath with your chin on your chest, simply makes you tired and makes your shoulders ache. It cuts off the supply of oxygen to your uterine muscles and to your baby. It doesn't get a baby born. Doing the breathing and worrying that you're not allowed to push if you feel the urge to bear down can also make you tense up, which is not helpful. So do the down breathing, and then just follow your body. Remember, you're the expert. Your brain may not know what to do if it is your first baby, but your body does. Remember, women in a coma have given birth.

If you have had an induced labour you may need to be guided when to push because the epidural may not have worn off fully so you can't feel for yourself what your body is telling you. This means you may be breathing your baby down less efficiently and you are more likely to need the help of an episiotomy, forceps or ventouse for your baby to be born.

In the past, a woman who had been coached when to push was then told to pant as the head passed through the pelvis and crowned. This is not necessary with KGH and is even intrusive because you have not been doing forced pushing in the first place. When you are relaxed and in a position that facilitates birth, you just continue with your relaxation and down breathing as your baby is born.

## Silence!

It's in the down stage of labours that midwives tend to start to talk and maintain a running commentary which is supposed to be encouraging. They have been taught to keep the mum cheerful and distracted during labour. KGH mums are different. You have knowledge about birth and how to facilitate it that is not the case for most women, and your midwife might not be accustomed to this. Politely ask your midwife to be completely silent. The reason is that, when someone talks to you it disturbs your peace of mind, and this stimulates the production of adrenaline. As we have already seen, adrenaline inhibits the production of oxytocin, the hormone needed to facilitate the working of the uterine muscles, the muscles needed to birth your baby. Women have commented that labour became more painful when the midwife started to talk because your body becomes less efficient. A polite explanation of this is in order to make sure your body is free to work efficiently and more comfortably.

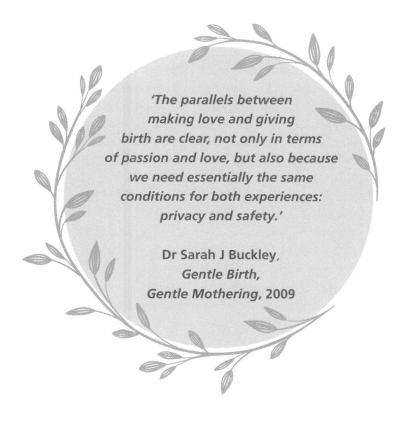

'The parallels between making love and giving birth are clear, not only in terms of passion and love, but also because we need essentially the same conditions for both experiences: privacy and safety.'

Dr Sarah J Buckley,
*Gentle Birth,*
*Gentle Mothering,* 2009

## Benefits of a vaginal birth

The down stage of labour puts pressure on the baby which is thoroughly beneficial. It is like a really powerful massage. It stimulates the baby's circulation, flexes muscles and helps to clear the lungs of mucus. Knowing this can be quite encouraging for fathers, particularly first-time fathers who may not have held a newborn baby before and might be afraid they could crush it or break its ribs. When you consider the pressure a baby has been under during the birth process, just picking up a baby normally is never going to hurt it.

Also, while in the womb, your baby's nutrition has been provided by you through the placenta and the cord rather than through its own digestive system. During a vaginal birth the baby picks up its mother's microorganisms, to which it already has its mother's immunity, and its gut flora begins to be quickly established. This forms the basis of its immune system. So everything has been thought of. It is a perfectly balanced, almost miraculous process, and the more I see of it, the more I am in awe of the miracle of birth. After birth the sense of smell is important in the bonding of mother and baby. In its passage through the birth canal a baby learns to recognise its mother's smell, which helps it to recognise her once it is born.

Women sometimes wonder how anything the size of a small melon (a baby's head) can fit through a passage the size of a vagina. The answer is that a woman's body, would you believe it, is designed to give birth. If that were not the case, the human race would not have survived. The vagina does not only stretch but also unfolds. If you think of a polo neck sweater, it becomes shorter as you stretch it wider to pull it over your head. The vagina is similar, in that the birth canal becomes shorter as the baby passes through it. The hormones of birth increase the flexibility of the tissue so it expands more easily. It's not the only sexual organ that changes shape and size when performing the function it is designed to do. It would be strange if it were otherwise. Also the plates of the baby's head are not yet formed so they can overlap. If you see a picture of the shape of a baby's head during birth, it is a quite extraordinary shape, longer and narrower than after it is born. A woman's pelvis is not one single bone, but several bones joined together by cartilage which becomes more flexible at the time of birth. All these things combine to facilitate a your baby's passage into the world.

Women have sometimes been a little concerned about opening their bowels when they get the urge to push. It can feel a little similar, and we are programmed not to open our bowels in public and maybe to feel a bit embarrassed by it. This concern can even slow down or stall labour. The first thing to understand is that it is almost impossible. In the last few weeks of pregnancy, when the baby's head has engaged, there is considerable competition for space in the pelvis and the capacity of the bowel and also the bladder is much reduced. There simply isn't room. This is why you may need to get up in the night in late pregnancy to go to the toilet. As the baby's head moves down during labour, it pushes the contents of the bowel and the bladder in front of it so you will want to go to the toilet more frequently, and, as the head passes through the birth canal, it completely closes the rectum and the urethra so it would be impossible for anything to get out of the bowel or the bladder at that point. There may be a very small amount of faecal matter pushed out in front of the baby's head. Midwives are quite used to this and you will be completely unaware and won't notice it even if it does happen. The midwife will simply scoop it out of the pool and dispose of it. In fact it is a welcome sign for midwives as it means the baby's head is about to emerge and your baby will be born very soon.

As a tiny example of the miracle of birth and how everything is linked to and co-ordinated with everything else, the passage through the birth canal is a time of pressure and stress for the baby. During each surge the baby's heartbeat may slow a little because of the pressure it is under. The midwife will check the baby's heartbeat after each surge to make sure it has returned to normal. Women are sometimes worried if they hear someone say that the baby's heart has slowed during a surge, but this is normal, and the midwife is interested in the recovery after the surge. As a result of this pressure the baby produces cortisol, the hormone of stress. When the baby is born the cortisol triggers the release of surfactant, lubricant, in its lungs which facilitates the lungs opening out and starting to function when the baby needs to breathe for itself. So the stress during birth and the release of cortisol is actually part of the process that established normal breathing through the lungs after birth. The more I learn of things like this, the more I am in awe of the process of birth, and understand that you disturb the natural process at your peril unless there is a very definite clinical reason. Watching a normal birth unfold is a humbling experience.

## *Takeaways*

* Courteously ask your midwife to be silent during the down stage of labour and offer a polite explanation.

* Down breathing focuses your body and mind downwards, as your baby moves down through the birth canal.

* Use your down breathing and also your soft and open images and visualisations to help you.

* You will know whether you want to bear down, or whether the down breathing and visualisations are sufficient on their own.

* Vaginal birth equips your baby well for life in the world; it stimulates the circulation, clears the lungs, massages muscles, introduces microorganisms that colonise the gut and form the basis of its immune system. It is truly miraculous.

# CHAPTER 22

# The Golden Hour

And then your baby is born! Words can't describe it! One father said:

> 'Words can't describe how I feel, and no-one who has never had a baby will ever understand.'

And that is the very best description I have ever heard. You didn't know before that love like this even existed, and you have never felt this quality of love before.

The first hour is a very important hour of your baby's life, which is why it is called the golden hour. Do read the book, *Birthing Your Placenta: The Third Stage of Labour* by Nadine Edwards and Sara Wickham so that you have the facts about this significant part of birth and understand the choices you need to make.

You may not have considered what happens in the hour after the baby is born, but this is a significant time in its development and its establishment in the world and you need to be well-informed so you can make your choices. It is one of the most important hours of your baby's life and a time for bonding for your new small family. It should be treated with the greatest respect.

## Skin-to-skin contact

We can't begin to imagine the shock of coming into this world; but we do know that the only things a newborn baby recognises are its mother's skin, the rhythm of its mother's breathing and heartbeat, its mother's and father's voices, and also its mother's smell, which it has learnt to recognise during the birth process. So it is very important for your baby to get back to these as quickly as possible.

A newborn baby doesn't need to be wiped, taken by a midwife, checked, weighed, or anything else. It needs mum – NOW! The most important thing is ideally for you to pick up your baby and hold it straight to your chest – no hesitations, but straight onto the chest for skin-to-skin contact. A baby will tend to settle comfortably as soon as it is in its mother's arms. It will be the same weight at the end of the golden hour, and any checks can be done just as easily while it is in your arms.

It may open its eyes and search for your face, and this is part of its natural brain development. If the light is too bright, it won't want to open its eyes, rather like being woken up by the sun shining in your face on a summer's morning, so it is better to welcome your baby into a dimly lit room which is a more gentle arrival into the world. This is why it is suggested that you have the lights dimmed in your half of theatre in the event of needing a Caesarean.

Babies that have an hour's skin-to-skin contact straight after birth tend to start to feed naturally during this time. Many babies lose weight for a couple of days after birth and then start to put on weight and grow. KGH babies often start to put on weight straight away as they have not had a trauma to recover from. If your baby is skin-to-skin on your chest, it stays warmer too as your body increases the blood supply to the chest where you are holding your baby to keep it warm, and a warm baby is more likely to start being interested in feeding, which he or she will demonstrate by licking or nuzzling at the breast and nipple, or by trying to locate the nipple, sometimes by turning their head when they feel a touch on the cheek. These normal responses tend to work best when the baby is skin-to-skin with the mother so that other reflexes (such as putting their fists in their mouth and sucking them) tend to be switched off. Within about 20 minutes of birth, a baby with skin-to-skin contact will tend to naturally find the nipple on its own, just like other mammals, and it is the gentlest and most supportive entrance into this new world. In the UK we are lucky because skin-to-skin for the baby on the mother's chest for at least an hour is universal practice. You can see examples of the 'breast crawl', when a baby finds the nipple on its own, on the internet.

It is also important for the mother to be kept warm after birth. You may find you are quite shivery and cold so it is important that your partner is ready to turn up the heating if you give birth at home. Mum being cold after birth can be a contributory factor in a retained placenta.

If there is a reason why the mother can't hold her baby all the time – perhaps after a Caesarean section, though this is unusual – then the baby can have skin-to-skin contact with the partner instead, and there is still the rhythm of breathing and a heartbeat. There is still a voice that it knows. You will both be smelling the delightful scent of your new baby, and the baby will be 'programming' you to love and nurture it by this clever scent message.

You might consider not telling family members when you go into labour (unless they are your birth partner, of course) or when the baby is born until you have had that first special hour together. If you have told them when you go into labour you will be aware at the most subtle level that they are longing to know about progress and whether the baby has arrived, and this is subconscious stress for you. They might even be sending your partner a surreptitious message to find out about progress. And that privacy of that first special hour after birth is very important and just for you. Welcome your wider family's congratulations and celebrations after that hour, but even then, you might like to ask them to respect your need for privacy. It is a special time for the new little family to bond together and get to know each other.

## Optimal cord cutting

When your baby is born it will still be attached by the umbilical cord to the placenta. The cord will continue to pulsate for a few minutes because the baby's blood will still be passing through it to the placenta, where it picks up oxygen and nutrients, and returns with them to the baby. Nature is clever and has ensured that, for a short time after birth, your baby is still connected to the life support system it has had for the last nine months, at the same time as it starts to breathe for itself – so it has a dual support system for a few minutes. About a third of the baby's blood is in the cord and placenta at any time, so if you cut the cord instantly at birth, you are depriving the baby of up to a third of its blood. I have been told that early cord clamping and cutting can be detected in the composition of the baby's blood for three or even six months after birth. How would you feel if you were suddenly deprived of about a third of your blood? I have been told that, if you give blood, you are only allowed to give a maximum of 8 per cent of your blood at any time. We have been routinely depriving our babies of 30 per cent of their blood for many years. If that happened to you it would take you weeks to recover. It's no wonder babies have sometimes taken a while to recover from the process of birth.

With the medicalisation of birth, it became normal to clamp and cut the umbilical cord immediately after birth. There was no evidence to justify this intervention, no research into the repercussions and benefits, nobody asked questions or thought it through properly. How many more interventions does this apply to? We now realise that it is of great benefit to wait until the cord has finished pulsating before clamping and cutting it, which means that all the baby's blood is back in its body. Even if you wait a minute it is an improvement on instant cord clamping, and three minutes is even better. The current guidelines in the UK advocate delayed cord clamping of 1 to 3 minutes, which is better than doing it immediately, though this is sometimes interpreted as 1 minute. After all, healthcare professionals are busy people. The guidelines specifically say that this applies to Caesareans as well. It is better still to wait until the cord has finished pulsating, which generally doesn't last long. You can see when this has happened or, to be sure, feel it. The phrase which is used as a guide is 'wait for white' as the cord is red when it has blood in it and it goes white when all your baby's blood is safely back in its body. Indeed, the latest research shows that it is even better for the baby to wait until the placenta has been expelled before the cord is cut, as the stem cell count in the baby increases dramatically if you wait. A few hospitals have already adopted this procedure.

Some couples opt for a 'lotus birth' where the baby is not separated from its placenta at birth. The cord is a jelly-like substance called Wharton's jelly which has been in the amniotic fluid during pregnancy. As soon as it comes out into the atmosphere it starts to dry out so, after a day or so, it shrivels up and can be pulled apart. It doesn't need to be clamped because there is no longer any blood in it, and it has been observed that the stump of the cord separates from the baby's naval sooner after a lotus birth than if the cord has been clamped and cut.

To read more about how important this is go to the websites: waitforwhite.com or bloodtobaby.com

## The placenta

One benefit of immediate breastfeeding is that breastfeeding is nipple stimulation, which encourages the production of oxytocin, and oxytocin is the hormone that makes the uterine muscles work, so this helps to expel the placenta.

Probably no-one has told you, but it is helpful to know in advance, that your surges will continue after your baby is born in order to expel the placenta. It can be disconcerting to feel the surges, gentler surges, continue after your baby has been born if you don't expect it. Indeed, gentle surges will go on for several days or even weeks after your baby is born as you breastfeed, and this could be nature's way of helping your muscles get back to normal and your tummy to get flat again after the birth of your baby. Maybe it is nature's way of rewarding you for breastfeeding. So everything links in miraculously with everything else and a breastfeeding mother is likely to get her tummy flat quicker.

There will also be bleeding after the birth while the area where the placenta was attached heals. This bleeding is like a heavy period and will go on for longer than a period does. It could continue for two or three weeks, or even up to a month, but it will be reducing all the time and is perfectly normal. It happens to everyone, and I'm telling you now so you know what to expect.

Your body has done the most amazing and flexible stretch during pregnancy so you need to understand that it does take a while to return to normal. You may need to continue to wear your maternity clothes or other loose clothes for a while after birth. But it is good to have been told this in advance rather than it coming as a disappointing shock at the time. Raspberry leaf tea, breast feeding, pelvic floor exercises and the exercises suggested by your physiotherapist will help you regain your figure.

The placenta is generally expelled within about 30 minutes after birth. As with everything to do with birth and babies, this length of time is simply an indication and can be very different. A placenta can arrive after ten minutes, half an hour, an hour, two hours. Sometimes the expulsive urge as you go to the toilet will help it drop out.

I will tell you a story about a suspected 'retained placenta'. As well as the NICE guidelines, local trusts issue further guidelines to their midwives, including when to transfer to hospital from a homebirth for a manual removal of the placenta in the event of a 'retained placenta'. Guidelines in maternity services tend to be regarded as rules.

In this case, the placenta had not arrived within the specified time and the midwife, quite correctly said, 'If your placenta hasn't arrived within two contractions, we ought to transfer into hospital for a manual removal.' Think for a moment what this will do to the mother. She will feel stressed and alarmed. What happens when a mum is stressed and alarmed? She produces the hormone adrenaline which inhibits the production of oxytocin, the hormone needed to make the uterine muscles work. Is it likely that she will expel her placenta within the next two contractions? No.

The wonderful doula who was also an excellent KGH teacher said, 'I know what I'll do. I'm going to get a blanket and make a tent. You and your husband can snuggle up inside the tent with your baby and I'll read you a relaxation. At the end of the relaxation I'll simply say, "Now stand up, and birth your placenta with gravity".'

What was she achieving by this? She was giving them privacy. Oxytocin is a shy hormone that likes privacy. They are having a cuddle which feels good and brings comfort and calmness. The physical cuddle and the feel-good factor stimulate the production of oxytocin. What else? It's dark in that little tent. When it gets dark, we naturally produce the hormone melatonin, the hormone that helps us go to sleep each night when it gets dark. When we feel sleepy the mind becomes calm, and a calm mind stimulates the production of oxytocin. There are also melatonin receptors in the uterus, so in addition the production of melatonin helps the uterine muscles to work. Having the baby nuzzling at the breast is another way to produce oxytocin. Then the doula read the couple a relaxation, which calms the mind, and so produces yet more oxytocin. So what did this doula achieve? She created the best possible situation for the mother's body to produce the maximum oxytocin to enable the uterine muscles to work well and expel the placenta spontaneously.

So that was exactly what the doula did and, after she had read the relaxation, she simply said to the mother, 'Now stand up and birth your placenta with gravity', and she did.

This was wonderful care by the doula, and please note that the midwife had done nothing wrong, she was kind and supportive, and doing everything right according to the protocols and guidelines. The thing to note is that this is a wonderful example of the difference between imposing a result and facilitating a solution. Can you see the importance of this? This is the principle on which everything we have talked about in KGH is based. Throughout this book and throughout the KGH course our aim is to give you the knowledge and techniques to facilitate the gentle and natural birth you are planning, rather than imposing a solution.

Once you have had a gentle birth and are holding the whole world in your arms in the tiny body of your wonderful baby, you may not think much about the third stage of labour, the part of labour after the birth, and consider it simply a technicality to be completed as quickly as possible and the midwives will sort it all out. After all, the baby is born, and mother and baby are well, so what else is there to consider? But the third stage of labour, the golden hour, is a very important part of the process and, as in everything to do with birth, it is wise to treat it with respect and carefully consider your preferences. Huge changes are taking place in your baby's little body and it is one of the most important periods in your baby's life. So there are significant choices to be made.

The guidelines specify a managed third stage, so it is standard practice to give the mother an injection of synthetic oxytocin to help expel the placenta, but injecting oxytocin into the mother's circulation system inhibits the surge of natural oxytocin that a woman produces after giving birth. It is this natural surge of oxytocin that stimulates the release of the mothering and breastfeeding hormone in the mother's brain, including prolactin and also endorphins. The synthetic oxytocin makes the uterine muscles contract, so it is important the placenta is expelled from the uterus before it is fully contracted and a manual removal would become necessary. The midwife will apply cord traction to help bring the placenta out, but this can lead to a haemorrhage (post partum haemorrhage – PPH). The purpose of the injection is also to prevent blood loss, as the area where the placenta was attached is reduced.

One thing to consider is that after birth, a mother produces the biggest peak of oxytocin in her whole life. This hormone stimulates the release of a cocktail of hormones from the pituitary gland, which is an important part of the bonding of mother and baby, the stimulating of the mothering instinct, and the establishment of breastfeeding. Having an injection of synthetic oxytocin inhibits that natural peak of oxytocin which, like everything, is perfectly balanced in the miracle of birth. The injected oxytocin does not cross the mother's blood–brain barrier so it does not stimulate the release of hormones, and does this affect the bonding of mother and baby? There are those who believe it may, however, cross the baby's immature blood–brain barrier, and the effects of this are not known. Does it inhibit the baby's production of oxytocin that is designed to take place at the beginning of life? Does this affect its future production of oxytocin? How will this affect its relationships and its ability to love? All questions considered in the deeply perceptive book *The Scientification of Love* by Dr Michel Odent.

If you prefer to have a natural (physiological) third stage, the midwife will have the injection to hand and can immediately use it in the unlikely event of a haemorrhage.

Please note that, if you have had synthetic oxytocin during labour, which will be the case if your labour was induced, your body will no longer be producing natural oxytocin so you will need the synthetic oxytocin to stimulate muscular contractions in the uterus to expel the placenta.

## Vitamin K

The other thing that is offered at birth is vitamin K for the baby. Vitamin K is one of the main clotting factors in blood, and the vitamin K level in a newborn baby's blood is much lower than in adults. We do not know why this is the case. There is a theory that it may be because the blood needs to be thinner to reach the brain during the pressure the baby's head is under during birth, or that the blood needs to be thinner to circulate in the newborn baby's tiny capillaries to suffuse the organs, and particularly the lungs, which need to start working on their own account. We simply don't know.

So an injection is offered to bring the level of vitamin K in the baby's blood up to the adult level. This injection actually raises the level of vitamin K in the baby's blood above the adult level. It is given to prevent haemorrhage, in particular brain haemorrhage. The vitamin K can also be administered orally in three doses to ensure patient compliance. I am told it tastes horrible, so babies do their best to spit it out.

Brain haemorrhage in newborn babies is extremely rare, but it can cause brain damage or even death. This occurs in 1 in 11,000 babies, but we do not know if these babies had a pre-existing condition, were premature, or labour was induced, and the numbers are so small that it is difficult to do meaningful research. We do  know that, if antibiotics have been administered to the mother during labour, this risk may be slightly increased. It is given the label VKDB, Vitamin K Deficiency Bleeding, but it does seem a little strange to label all babies as deficient in vitamin K when they are naturally born that way. The injection is designed to prevent late onset VKDB, which extremely occasionally happens a couple of weeks after birth, so there is plenty of time to consider whether or not you want to have it for your baby. As with any intervention, take your time and consider the evidence in advance. An excellent source of information is Sara Wickham's book, *Vitamin K and the Newborn*. If you decide not to have the injection, make sure you are well informed what signs to look for and what action you would take in the unlikely event of any concern.

There is no research that indicates the injection does harm to babies. There is vitamin K in colostrum, the milk that a mother produces in the first few days of her baby's life. And if a mother eats a diet rich in vitamin K — which is found mainly in green, leafy vegetables — her breast milk will be richer in vitamin K, but this is not sufficient to bring the baby's level of vitamin K up to the same level as the injection. This is another subject that you need to read about in order to make an informed choice. Again, I would suggest the book *Vitamin K and the Newborn* by Sara Wickham which is an assessment of the facts and evidence. Once again you find yourself asking the question whether, except in very rare and unusual circumstances, we can trust that nature has got it right, or do we know better?

## DEVELOPING LIFE RELAXATION

It seems so long ago that this experience began and yet it is so immediate, too: the creation of new life in your body, deep within you, until the moment when you hold your baby in your arms. It seems like a true miracle, and indeed it is a miracle – the starting of life from nothing. And you are the person performing this miracle.

Your baby is already its own small person, moving and kicking inside you. Nature is bringing new life as she always does, and you are the person to receive this great gift as your baby slips gently into the world.

You are experiencing this, and the profound and life-enhancing changes it brings, and your baby too will change and develop in so many positive and delightful ways. These changes are the successful and happy result of these few months of pregnancy.

Your positive and happy state of mind develops and grows as you absorb the knowledge that all is natural and right, and so you become more and more confident, serene and calm. And the more calm, the more serene and the more confident you become, the happier you are, and this beneficial and self-confirming cycle makes things better and better for you, and for your baby.

# Confidence in a gentle birth

We have talked a lot about practical things, so let's do another relaxation. Settle yourself comfortably and listen to your partner reading this to you, or quietly read it to yourself. Do a few breaths of the long, slow, up breathing before you start, and then just listen.

Enjoying this experience today helps you physically, mentally and emotionally, and in every way you become much stronger and more confident and powerful. That strength and confidence give you more natural energy, and increase your joy and anticipation of your baby's swift and gentle birth.

You feel so at peace, and completely calm and serene, in your body and in your mind. What you visualise will be, and you maintain this knowledge and confidence regardless of whatever any other person may say or suggest, because you know with certainty that your birthing experience will be natural and gentle. Follow your instincts. Have confidence in your inner wisdom.

Your birthing experience will be as you have decided, as you have determined, as you have affirmed to yourself. It will be calm, serene and empowering as your body goes naturally through the miraculous process of giving birth to your baby. Nothing at all could be more wonderful than experiencing the miracle of birth.

As your body eases your baby gently into the world, and into your arms, the lessons you have learnt help you to move deeper and deeper into complete serenity and calm. Your body, your mind and your baby are all working together

*Continued overleaf...*

... *Continued from page 303*

in perfect harmony, so that all proceeds smoothly and naturally. Your mind is calm and serene. Everything is happening so calmly and smoothly.

You release gently and confidently as your body softens and opens. Your baby joins you in this natural and wonderful process, and you both instinctively act together at this very special time, your breath easing and slowing, deep and comfortable, your baby slipping gently into the world where you are waiting patiently and happily to hold your newborn infant.

This is a great natural process and nature knows exactly what to do. Nature creates the surges that flow and ebb in your body like the waves of the sea. Surges, ebbs, flows, all carry you along like the tides on the seashore, like the wash of the sea on the sand. You are carried along by these images; you breathe in harmony with them slowly, deeply and gently. As the sea washes and smooths the sand, so your body is calmed by its own natural, powerful drug, endorphins – completely in harmony with nature, your baby and your own body so completely at ease.

All is well. All is very well.

As the experience deepens so you deepen in it too, and the deeper you go the more serene you become, the easier and calmer your breathing is, the more your body follows its natural rhythms, and the more your baby joins with you in its smooth passage into the world.

Release, release, all is well, all is gentle, and all is so natural. Allow your body and thoughts to flow with the tide and be carried along in confidence and serenity towards the moment of your baby's birth.

See now that moment arrive. See now your baby coming

into the world. See now, where before your body held your baby in safety and comfort, now your arms hold your baby in warmth and love, and your baby's eyes open wide and gaze into yours.

This is the culmination of those special months of joyful anticipation, of preparing. Now you have brought your baby into the world naturally and lovingly. You always knew you could do it – and you have. You always knew it would happen like this.

You are both so happy and proud as you rest with your baby enfolded in your arms.

All is well.

## Takeaways

* Skin-to-skin contact immediately following birth is important and this is the natural start to breastfeeding. Wiping, weighing and measuring can all wait, and first checks can be done with your baby in your arms.

* Optimal (not just 'delayed') cord clamping and cutting is best for your baby. It needs its full quota of blood.

* The placenta will be expelled in its own time after the birth of your baby. The surges will continue to facilitate this.

* Be well informed about vitamin K so you can make the choice you feel comfortable with for your baby.

* Consider carefully whether you want a managed or physiological third stage of labour (the golden hour).

* Use the 'Developing Life' relaxation to help you to prepare for a calm and confident birth.

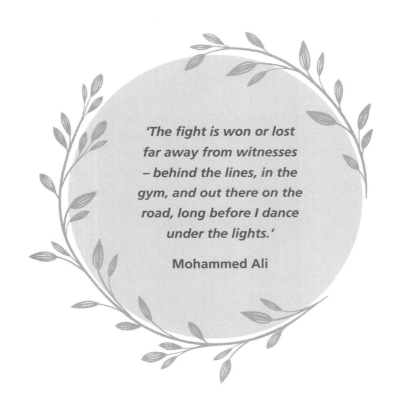

'The fight is won or lost far away from witnesses – behind the lines, in the gym, and out there on the road, long before I dance under the lights.'

Mohammed Ali

# CHAPTER 23

# Practising For the Birth You Want

K GH works. I have seen it time and time again. By letting go of the fear, negative thoughts and preconceptions you may have about childbirth, you allow the perfect system which is already created in your body to work efficiently and comfortably. Practice is paramount.

You are focused on a calm and natural birth, so it is very much in your best interests to carefully consider the aspects of birth we have talked about in this book in advance.

## Birth plans

A birth plan or birth proposal has two functions. First, it helps you to define your own ideas and encourages you to research the alternatives so you can choose wisely. Second, it tells your midwife how you would like her to support you during labour.

Midwives are busy people, and they will not have time to read three closely typed sheets of paper, so make your birth plan succinct. Cut out the waffle, the 'I really hope that' and 'If it were possible'. If you put the majority of it as bullet points on a single sheet of paper so that she can see at a glance exactly what you do and do not want, it will make her life much easier and mean that you are more likely to get what you want. Write the most important points at the top of the list so she sees them first. Your midwife wants to support you, so make it easy for her.

## BIRTH PROPOSAL TEMPLATE

Here is a list of all the aspects of childbirth we have looked at in this book. It is not a birth proposal, but you can use it as a checklist when you are writing your own birth proposal. It's a good idea to start with an acknowledgement that birth is a natural and unpredictable process and a note that, although these are your carefully considered wishes, you are willing to change your plans if necessary – on the basis of evidence-based advice:

I understand that this proposal may need to be changed according to clinical changes in the course of labour and the health needs of me and my baby. Please give me and my partner the evidence if a change is suggested.

WE WOULD LIKE:
☐ Give birth at home / in MLU / in OU
☐ Respect and support for our KGHypnobirthing
☐ Monitoring after 42 weeks rather than induction of labour
☐ A place of birth that supports privacy and calm and a natural birth
☐ Peace, tranquility and silence in my room
☐ Facility to play our KGH audio
☐ Any conversation to be with my partner in the first instance
☐ Positive language around me at all times
☐ Respect for the fact that conversation with mother disturbs the neocortex and stimulates the production of adrenalin which inhibits the production of oxytocin and so can make labour longer and more uncomfortable
☐ Support for me to take my position of choice during the birth
☐ My partner to remain with me throughout labour and birth and after the birth
☐ Private time with my partner to discuss any proposed procedure
☐ Use of the pool during labour and birth. (As KGH births can be quicker than other births please make sure the pool is filled in good time.)

PHYSIOLOGICAL THIRD STAGE:
- ☐ Immediate skin-to-skin – no wiping, weighing or checking of the baby first
- ☐ Partner to cut the cord
- ☐ Optimal cord clamping and cutting – wait for white (after pulsation has stopped and the placenta has been expelled)
- ☐ Lotus birth
- ☐ No injection of synthetic oxytocin at or after birth except in the event of post-partum haemorrhage (not prophylactically)
- ☐ Allow whatever time is needed for natural expulsion of the placenta
- ☐ Immediate skin-to-skin contact at birth and to continue for a full hour with no interruption
- ☐ Facilitate my baby to initiate breast feeding when it is ready at or after birth. Support to be available if asked for
- ☐ No infant feed supplements (cow's milk formula) to be given to my baby at any time, even at night
- ☐ Baby to receive vitamin K by injection / orally / not at all

WE PREFER NOT TO HAVE:
- ☐ Vaginal examinations
- ☐ Induction by membrane sweep
- ☐ Medical induction for length of pregnancy
- ☐ Any augmentation of labour
- ☐ Artificial rupture of membranes
- ☐ Vaginal examination after release of membranes
- ☐ In the event of release of membranes before surges start, we decline induction of labour and antibiotics
- ☐ Augmentation of labour: I agree to one vaginal examination at the beginning of labour
- ☐ The use of the word 'pain' in labour
- ☐ Conversation in my room throughout labour
- ☐ Any commentary or instruction during the second stage of labour. Silence would be very much appreciated

IN THE EVENT OF AN UNPLANNED CAESAREAN I WOULD LIKE:
- ☐ A relaxation script before entering theatre
- ☐ Gown worn back to front so chest left bare for skin-to-skin with baby
- ☐ Oximeter to be attached to my toe or non-dominant hand
- ☐ Monitoring leads to be placed on the side of my chest so I can easily hold my baby.
- ☐ My KGH audio to be played in theatre
- ☐ Lights dimmed in my half of theatre
- ☐ Screen to be dropped so I can see my baby being born
- ☐ Surgeon to make the incision and 'walk the baby out'
- ☐ Immediate skin to skin – no wiping, weighing or checking of baby first
- ☐ Optimal cord clamping and cutting – a lotus birth may be needed to facilitate this
- ☐ No taking baby to NICU as routine or prophylactically
- ☐ Baby and mother to be kept together at all times

If you decline certain aspects of care considered routine (vaginal examinations, for example, or a sweep or other form of induction of labour), the midwife has to be able to put 'mother declined' in the notes and have documented evidence of this. As we said before, it is best to sort out this in advance as you don't want to be having this conversation during labour, but include it in your birth proposal just to be sure. You can also have it put in your notes that you already had this conversation, you understood the advice you were given, and you do not agree to have it again. Always with the proviso, of course, that there is not a change in your clinical situation. Length of pregnancy is not a clinical change.

Midwives want to support you, and most will do their best to follow your birth proposal. Sometimes this doesn't happen, and your partner needs to be aware of your plan so they can gently nudge the midwife in the direction you want.

## Daily practice

Here is the simple and clear list that defines your practice. Your practice is important, but it needs to be done in a way that works for you so may need minor modifications to suit you and your lifestyle.

The practice suggested takes only 10–15 minutes a day, as asking anyone to practise for two hours a day would be unrealistic and simply wouldn't happen. If you are able to do more, perhaps once you are on maternity leave, that would be even better. You practise so that, by the time you use the breathing, visualisations and relaxations in labour, they are second nature and are deeply embedded in your subconscious mind. This will make them far more effective.

You have the upward breathing, the one you use during surges and also for practice, with the visualisations of the sun rising, blowing bubbles, or anything with an 'up' emphasis to facilitate the muscles that are working to draw up. You also have the soft and open visualisations to facilitate the cervix in thinning and opening. A few of these breaths, morning, and evening or whenever suits you, is all you need. You will find you naturally begin to use this breathing if ever you are stressed. It is a useful life-skill that can be used at other times and will remain with you after your baby is born.

There's the downward breathing to include from about Week 36. Do it with your partner so that you can practise the visualisations, but you can practise it on the toilet as well.

Next on the practice list are the relaxation scripts. Choose the one you like best for your partner to read to you before you go to bed each night:

- **Sssoften Relaxation** (page 70)
- **Stroking Relaxation** (page 72)
- **Calming Touch Relaxation** (page 74)

■ **Garden of Pregnancy Relaxation** (page 76)
■ **You Are in Control Relaxation** (page 79)

You can get these scripts on an audio as well:

■ **Garden of Pregnancy Relaxation**
■ **Play the *Ultimate Birth Relaxation* audio** as you go to sleep each night. This contains the Magic Carpet relaxation, the positive birth affirmations, and the Colour and Calmness relaxation.
■ **You can choose to listen to an individual audio** or have them all played consecutively.
■ **The lovely Confident and Positive relaxation as extra support.** (page 220)
■ **The 5Cs Relaxation** to help you release previous birth trauma. (page 164)
■ **The Gift of Bonus Time Relaxation** to help you remain happy and positive towards the end of your pregnancy (page 182)
■ **Include the gentle back stroking in your practice** – delicious!

All these practice items are for use as you give birth as well.

There are the pelvic floor exercises, which you incorporate into your lifestyle and do while you're waiting at red traffic lights or while the kettle boils for example. Once you have trained yourself for a couple of days you'll find yourself doing them automatically. Then they don't have to take extra time out of your busy and interesting life. Use the squeezy app if you find it helpful.

Perineal massage takes only five minutes from Week 36 when you will probably be on maternity leave.

Where practical, be in a more upright (or slightly forward)

DAILY PRACTICE

- Up breathing, with up and open images, for a few minutes morning and evening
- Down breathing, with down and open images from week 36 (also when on the loo)
- Have your partner read you a script each evening before bed: Sssoften Relaxation, Stroking Relaxation, Calming Touch Relaxation, or Garden of Pregnancy Relaxation
- Confident and Positive Relaxation or The Gift of Bonus Time Relaxation from week 40
- Listen to the *Colour and Calmness* audio as you go to sleep: The Magic Carpet Relaxation, Positive Birth Affirmations, and The Colour and Calmness Relaxation
- Confident and Positive Relaxation or The 5Cs Relaxation whenever helpful
- Gentle back stroking

Also:

- Put up positive birth affirmations around your home. Change their position from time to time to maintain interest
- Pelvic floor exercises
- Perineal massage from week 36
- Being more upright to encourage your baby into the most usual position
- Look at the picture of the baby in the most usual position for birth

Practise, practise, practise.
Focus your attention on where you want to be.
Position and relaxation are the most important things.

position to encourage your baby to be in the most usual position facing your back, ready for birth.

Then there's the birth picture to look at frequently. The body follows where the mind leads, and this picture puts a positive image of your baby's position in your mind and looking at it takes no time at all. Put it somewhere prominent in your home and remember to notice it as you go past.

One very important thing is to focus your attention on where you want to be. If anything distracts you from it, set aside the distraction and resume your focus – because what you focus on is what you get. This daily practice only takes about 10–15 minutes; 20 minutes at the most when you include the perineal massage.

Remember also to prepare about half a dozen funny movies. Prepare your schedule for bonus time.

## Practice is essential

For a successful KGH experience, it is vital to practise the breathing, visualisations and relaxations during your pregnancy. It will make a difference to your life. The reports I receive from hypnobirthing mothers show that it was the couples' practice that made all the difference as well as making choices based on facts and not on fear:

*We worked together almost daily before the birth on visualisations and listening to the audios before bed.*

*The whole experience was beautiful because my husband and I made it that way.*

*I put a large amount of effort into the practice I did at home, listening to your audio, reading aloud my affirmations and doing the relaxation exercises every day for two and a half months without fail. As a direct result I had not only the birth that I wanted, I had the perfect birth.*

*I was terrified from the day I realised I was pregnant.*

*I joined your course, did the homework, and tried to relax as much as possible. I guess all the work I did paid off. I am sure it would have been a completely different story if I hadn't joined your course.*

## When your baby is coming:

- **Use the Confident and Positive script**
- **Take your time, conserve your energy,** gently keep doing what you were doing
- **If possible have a massage or reflexology,** etc.
- **Have a rest**
- **Start timing your surges**
- **Watch a funny movie**
- **Take a warm bath**
- **Use your up breathing**
- **Play the Colour and Calmness audio**
- **Snack to keep your energy up**
- **Remember to sip water so you keep dehydrated**
- **Call the midwife** when your surges are 3-4 minutes apart and one minute long and regular

## Using KGH throughout the birth

For you, the mother, throughout the birth all there is to do is the up breathing with the up visualisations, moving to the down breathing and the down and open visualisations. It's that simple. You may find one of the prompts or positive statements comes to mind like a mantra.

Your positive colour and image of a beautiful pink rose will be there to support you.

Mothers sometimes worry because usually, if there's something important in your life such as an exam, you revise for it as much as possible, you cram in more and more, and then you produce it on the day. KGHypnobirthing is exactly the opposite. All your practice is to let go. The more you practise the more you let go and release, and release and let go of assumptions, preconceptions, stresses, worries, etc, so that, by the time you give birth to your baby, there is nothing left to inhibit the perfect system, which is your body and mind working in the way they are designed to do. The system created within you is a shining diamond of perfection and you couldn't possibly improve on it. You do all the practice and you have no way of checking how well it works until you give birth – and it does.

Your partner is the guardian of your impenetrable bubble of peace and positivity. Your partner's role is to protect your space – physically, mentally and emotionally – and be your advocate. It is very helpful if your partner can come with you to antenatal visits, particularly in the later stages of pregnancy, because nature programmes you mentally and emotionally to go into your own space ready for birth, so you may need someone with you to have a conversation on your behalf that you could perfectly well have had yourself a few weeks previously.

Your partner also has the role of giving you gentle prompts during your surges if you find that helpful; reading relaxation scripts if appropriate; gently stroking your back or arms, or anywhere that is convenient; and playing the *Ultimate Birth Relaxation* audio for you. It's also important to make sure you always have water available to sip with a few drops of Five Flower Remedy in it, and with a drinking straw so you don't have to change position every time you take a sip.

Your partner could also make sure essential oil of lavender is available for you to help you relax; give you arnica pills to support the tissue; and make sure a selection of light snacks is available in case you feel like eating.

- **Remain calm and confident.**
- **Allow your birthing body to birth your baby.**
- **Birthing and caring for your baby is a natural process of being.**

## Whatever you do is right

The fact that you have read this book shows you are caring parents. Every parent brings up their child in a different way. Every parent, before their baby is born, thinks they are going to bring it up in a particular way, and then after it is born, they realise that the child is already its own person, and your role as a parent is simply to support him or her in every way you can, to give them all the opportunities you can, and then, when you see which way they want to go, to run along behind, trying to keep up as they develop.

It is the most wonderful and important thing that you can do in life, and you must always remember that whatever choices you make and whatever you do is right. There is no such thing as a perfect parent. Every parent will look back and feel guilty about something they should or shouldn't have done, or could or couldn't have done. But the important thing for your child is your love.

## Resource sheets

We have produced a number of free resource sheets for you covering many of the aspects of birth or the choices you will need to make that may concern you.

These can be downloaded for free from the KGH website: kghb.org/sheets. You will find the list of these very useful sheets at the back of this book. The Resource Sheets are being added to and updated in the light of the latest research all the time. You can always find the most recent version at kghb.org/sheets.

The available sheets will address the key points of many of the situations you may find yourself in throughout your pregnancy and at the birth of your baby. If there is another one that would be helpful, let us know, and we will look into producing it for you. If you feel the need for it, it's very likely that other women will too.

'Do good without show or fuss, Facilitate what is happening rather than what you think ought to be happening, If you must take the lead, lead so that the mother is helped, yet still free and in charge. When the baby is born, the mother will rightly say: We did it ourselves.'

Lao Tzu

## THE RIVER RELAXATION

Here is a last relaxation for you to enjoy:

Take three gentle, slow, deep breaths, then, as you quietly listen to my voice, I want to tell you that hypnosis is simply a learning experience, and we've all had so many learning experiences. For example, I once went boating on a river. This was a place and a time that was special to me, and as you listen you may find that you are drifting off to a place and time that was special to you, that had particular meaning for you. It all began when I found myself climbing from the bank into a wooden boat. I always wondered what it would be like to take a boat down the river to an island. Someone once told me that a beautiful flower grew there, and I always wondered what it would be like.

I set off, not knowing what the experience would be like. I was a little apprehensive of not being on the solid land to which I was accustomed, but my closest friend and some other people who were experienced were with me and I felt reassured and comforted by their presence. I felt the boat rocking back and forth with each breath, rocking back and forth with each breath, as the current drew it into the middle of the river. I noticed that the river wasn't exactly straight, but wound through the vegetation. And I noticed all different kinds of trees. I saw the sunlight stream through the branches.

The sound of the water gurgling and splashing around me was soothing. I trailed my hand in the water and it felt cool and refreshing. It felt so good as I took a deep breath, and I realised I could just take my time. I decided to just enjoy the moment and took another deep breath, and I breathed deeply and comfortably. I realised that I could be

*Continued overleaf...*

*... Continued from page 319*

entirely confident: my boat was sturdy, and I was surrounded by people who would take care of me. There seemed to be a calmness as I wondered … I wondered what it would be like to reach the island and see the wonderful flower I was expecting to see.

So I just released and let the river carry me swiftly downstream … further and further. The air was so wonderful to breathe in, I filled my lungs … That's right … With each breath I took I became more and more at peace. It was a sunny day and I felt warm and comfortable. There was no need to move or talk, so I just allowed my eyes to close, so that I could fully enjoy the experience. And isn't it good to know that we can feel just as comfortable and at ease, even now? I felt so secure and peaceful that, sitting comfortably, I began to let go of all my worries and fears, all the tension, and simply began to increasingly release … all the way.

The river became wider and wider as it carried me to my destination, bringing me closer to my destination each time the current surged. So I just released and let go of any fears and tension. The river surged and slowed again, surging and slowing, surging then slowing, and each time I became more and more at peace, I was just happy that I was being carried … further and further … towards the end of my journey.

Finally the river ended in a small lake, and I was surprised how quickly I had reached the end of the river. In the middle of the lake was a beautiful island, full of wonderful plants and flowers. My boat was carried right to the shore of the island – all I had to do was release and allow the boat to be guided by the current. I was so excited, because I was finally going to see the wonderful flower that I had seen in my imagination so many times. I was finally going to see the flower blossom.

I got out of the boat and stepped onto the island. I could hear birdsong, and the sound of the water lapping against the shore. I could feel the gentle warmth of the sun on my back. I walked swiftly along a short, wide, grassy path to the centre of the island and there, in the very middle, was my flower. It was more beautiful than I had even imagined. I held the blossom in my hands, now gently opened into full bloom, and the petals felt so soft and tender as I inhaled its sweet fragrance.

I sat down nearby and just enjoyed the feeling of happiness and joy for a while. I found my mind wandering to very enjoyable, calm and peaceful times; times when I found that I was confident and strong; times when I trusted in my own body, and trusted in my subconscious to instinctively guide me; times when I felt filled with love and deep tranquillity, situations where I could allow this energy to flow through me – through every cell in my body. Really focused within me, aware of the strength within myself, of power, of confidence, and those things that we were never really taught as we grew up, I discovered that I could give myself all those things at that moment.

I took my time and enjoyed the feeling moving through my body and permeating every cell. That sense, that feeling that was always there – I just hadn't known it was there.

When I was ready and in my own time, I came back, bringing with me all that I had learned.

And now you can open your eyes and come back to the here and now.

*(Thank you, Moira Campbell, for permission to use this script.)*

## The benefit of KGH for your baby

As a mother, you have probably come to KGH for a calm, gentle birth for yourself, and this also means a calm and gentle birth for your baby.

Birth is the most formative experience of our lives, and a baby who enters the world drug-free and alert, to be greeted by a mother who is also alert, loving and confident, starts life and forms its first relationship in this world in the best possible way.

There is a serenity and poise about KGH babies which is difficult to define but frequently remarked upon and, from the reports I get from mothers years later, this special quality remains with the child as it grows and develops.

Though women come to KGHypnobirthing for a more comfortable birth for themselves, which it can certainly deliver, in the longer term the benefits for your baby could be even more significant.

Have a beautiful birth and a wonderful baby.

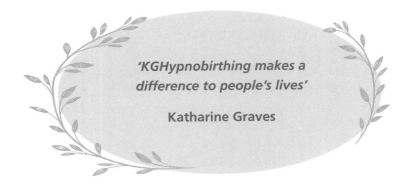

'KGHypnobirthing makes a difference to people's lives'

**Katharine Graves**

## Takeaways

* Make your choices logically and based on evidence.
* Ask questions.
* Trust your instinct.
* Use our sample Birth Proposal to help you to create your plan.
* Practise in pregnancy: I know we have said it before, but it is so important.
* All the practice you have done will be there for you when your baby is on its way.
* Continue to use your KGH techniques for relaxation throughout birth.
* Diana's birth story (page 276) shows how one mum actually used everything we have talked about when she gave birth.
* KGH is not just good for you, but is also beneficial for your baby. This is very important and, in the long term, possibly even more important than a more comfortable birth for you.
* Read the birth stories on the KGH website. You will enjoy them.
* Please leave a review kghb.org/review. This helps us to help other women to experience the positive birth which should be the experience of everyone giving birth.

## KGH Birth Stories

Go to the website kghb.org/birthreports where you will be able to read all the wonderful birth stories from mothers, fathers, partners and midwives. I hope they will inspire you.

# What to pack for hospital

Whether you are planning to have your baby at home or in hospital, it is worth getting together the things you may need.

---

### FOR THE MOTHER, FOR THE BIRTH

- ☐ Hospital notes
- ☐ Birth proposal
- ☐ Your KGH folder
- ☐ Your KGH positive birth cards
- ☐ *The Hypnobirthing Book*
- ☐ *Ultimate Birth Relaxation* audio
- ☐ Your relaxing colour
- ☐ Picture of beautiful pink rose
- ☐ Note to midwife
- ☐ Nightdress or pyjamas
- ☐ Large, old T-shirt to wear for the birth
- ☐ Snacks (e.g. bananas, cereal bars)
- ☐ Water
- ☐ Bendy drinking straws
- ☐ Dressing gown
- ☐ Slippers, socks
- ☐ Mobile phone and charger
- ☐ Laptop or tablet
- ☐ Magazine, book
- ☐ Tissues
- ☐ Essential oil of lavender
- ☐ Five Flower Remedy
- ☐ Arnica pills
- ☐ Your pillow
- ☐ Birthing ball *(check if your hospital has them)*
- ☐ Spare pillows in the car

---

## FOR THE MOTHER, AFTER THE BIRTH

- ☐ Maternity pads (2 packs)
- ☐ Plenty of big cotton pants
- ☐ 2 or 3 nursing bras
- ☐ Breast pads
- ☐ Aloe vera gel
- ☐ Nipple cream
- ☐ Stretch mark lotion
- ☐ Front-opening nightdress, pyjamas or shirt
- ☐ Toiletries, hairbrush, towels
- ☐ Clothes for going home *(you won't fit into your normal clothes yet)*

## FOR THE PARTNER

- ☐ Mobile phone and charger
- ☐ Camera
- ☐ Toiletries, including shaving gear for men
- ☐ Snacks
- ☐ Water
- ☐ Book
- ☐ Laptop or tablet *(but make sure they know they mustn't be tempted to play on it when you need their care and attention)*
- ☐ Swimwear *(if they are going to join you in the birthing pool)*
- ☐ Pyjamas *(if they can stay the night after the birth)*

## FOR THE BABY

- ☐ Nappies (allow 12 a day)
- ☐ 2 or 3 sleepsuits
- ☐ 2 or 3 vests
- ☐ Muslin squares
- ☐ Pair of socks or booties
- ☐ Suit for going home
- ☐ Jacket or snowsuit for winter babies
- ☐ Hat
- ☐ Car seat *(NB. taxis often only have seats for older babies, aged nine months and over)*

# Resources

## KGHypnobirthing classes

You can access the KGHypnobirthing course in different ways, from face-to-face in a group session to virtually from your own home. The online course is also available for you to stream and watch in your own time. You may be an expectant parent looking for techniques to help with a calm and comfortable birthing experience; maybe you are interested in training as a KGHypnobirthing teacher, perhaps already a midwife or doula looking to learn something new. This book will have helped a lot, but accessing the classes will take what you learn to the next level. Visit kghb.org/kghcourse for more details.

## FACE-TO-FACE CLASSES

Katharine personally teaches group classes in London where, in addition to the full KGH training, you can have your questions answered, and plenty of time for discussion, as well as the benefit of meeting other expectant parents. You can reserve a place on these classes at kghb.org/kghcourse.

Reading this book, and practising the relaxations is very effective, but there really is no substitute for a face-to-face KGHypnobirthing class. The interaction between you and your teacher, your own questions answered, and the full engagement of your partner all contribute to making a taught class the best option, offering the very best outcomes. It gives you the opportunity to practise the relaxations fully and cover all the necessary material in depth to gain the most benefit when giving birth.

KGHypnobirthing trained teachers offer classes throughout the UK and are taught in many countries around the world. All our teachers are fully trained and skilled in the delivery of KGH courses, and we couldn't recommend them more highly! But make sure the course you book on is the full 12-hour KGH antenatal training, otherwise you are getting less than the best and being short-changed.

## VIRTUAL CLASSES

Katharine also teaches virtual classes which you can find on the website kghb.org/kghcourse if you want to reserve your place. The virtual classes have the same content as the face-to-face course and have proved to be remarkably effective. You can join these classes from anywhere in the world.

## KGHYPNOBIRTHING ONLINE COURSES

It can sometimes be impractical or even impossible for you to attend a face-to-face KGHypnobirthing class, or there may not be a teacher near you.

It is so important that KGHypnobirthing is accessible to all expectant mothers and their partners as we want you to have the opportunity to fully benefit from a KGHypnobirthing course, so we have developed the complete KGHypnobirthing Online Course delivered by Katharine Graves and streamed direct to your home. The online course covers the same full content as the face-to-face course, all the expertise, advice and guidance you need, and you can re-watch any section to reinforce your knowledge. Find it at kghb.org/kgonline.

There is a Facebook group for you to join if you have done the online course, so you can ask questions, and talk to and meet other KGH couples.

**SOCIAL MEDIA**

 FACEBOOK

Please join our Hypnobirthing Group on Facebook at kghb.org/fb.
There is a wealth of experience here at your fingertips from midwives, hypnobirthing teachers and mums. So please ask questions, share your news and your experiences. We all love to read birth stories as well, so please pop back and share yours with us.

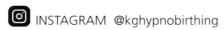 INSTAGRAM @kghypnobirthing

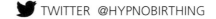 TWITTER @HYPNOBIRTHING

## KGHYPNOBIRTHING TEACHER TRAINING COURSES

For those interested in learning to become a KGH teacher, KGHypnobirthing offer the market-leading course accredited by the Royal College of Midwives.

More and more midwives are referring couples to KGHypnobirthing and the demand for classes is growing. Being able to teach with confidence the simplicity of a natural and calm birth to expectant mothers and their partners, is a privilege and is deeply satisfying.

This comprehensive training programme of choice for midwives appeals to midwives, doulas, mothers, hypnotherapists, doctors, nutritionists, and anyone who is interested in making a difference. It leads to the KGHypnobirthing diploma.

It is a privilege to be a hypnobirthing teacher, knowing that you are making a positive difference to a mother's experience of birth and to her baby's life.

These courses are offered face-to-face in the UK, and can be arranged elsewhere on request. We also offer virtual courses at different times so there is a convenient course for you in whatever time zone you may live. Find out more at kghb.org/teacher.

# Books

Here is a list of books that you might find helpful:

## ESSENTIAL READING

*The AIMS Guide to Induction of Labour*, Nadia Higson

## VERY IMPORTANT READING

*Group B Strep Explained*, Sara Wickham

*Birthing Your Placenta*, Nadine Edwards and Sara Wickham

*Gestational Diabetes*, Sara Wickham

*Why Caesarean Matters*, Clare Goggin

*Vitamin K And The Newborn*, Sara Wickham

## VERY USEFUL READING

*The AIMS Guide to Your Rights in Pregnancy & Birth*, Emma Ashworth

*Primal Health: Understanding the Critical Period Between Conception and the First Birthday*, Michel Odent

*Ina May's Guide to Childbirth*, Ina May Gaskin

*The Thinking Woman's Guide to a Better Birth*, Henci Goer

*Gentle Birth, Gentle Mothering: A Doctor's Guide to Natural Childbirth and Gentle Early Parenting Choices*, Sarah J. Buckley

*Breech Birth: A Guide to Breech Pregnancy and Birth*, Benna Waites

*The AIMS Guide to Twin Pregnancy and Birth*, Rebecca Freckleton

# Audios

The following audios can help you to achieve a calm and natural birth, and to enjoy a confident and happy pregnancy. They are all available from kghb.org/audios.

## ANTENATAL AUDIOS

*Ultimate Birth Relaxation* – your essential relaxation. The instructions to download this are at the beginning of this book.

*Confident and Positive Relaxation* – your daily pregnancy relaxations. Includes the Sssoften Relaxation, the Stroking Relaxation, and Calming Touch relaxation. Also the fear release and confidence building Confident & Positive relaxation.

*Knowledge and Reassurance* – your baby's breech birth

*Positive and Gentle* – your baby's Caesarean birth

*Armenian Lullaby* – Gurdjieff and de Hartman
The background music on all our audios and for use when you are practising at home.

## POSTNATAL AUDIOS

Do make a note of these. You will find them extremely supportive after your baby has arrived.

*Nurture and Nature* – breastfeeding your baby

*Self Belief* – caring for you as a new mum

*A Moment of Calm* – peace amidst the hurly burly of family life

## OTHER AUDIOS

*Relax and Conceive* – your effective aid to conception

# Useful websites

**KGHypnobirthing** www.kghypnobirthing.com
For hypnobirthing, a list of professional hypnobirthing teachers, teacher training courses, books and audios.

**Association for Improvements in the Maternity Services (AIMS)** www.aims.org.uk
Provides information on pregnancy and birth and a free helpline.

**Midwife Thinking** www.midwifethinking.com
Excellent factual and researched information about many aspects of pregnancy and birth.

**Sara Wickham** www.sarawickham.com
Draws together research and evidence about pregnancy and birth in an accessible form. An excellent source of information.

**Independent Midwives** www.im.org.uk
A wonderful group of midwives who have profound knowledge and experience of supporting physiological birth in many different circumstances.

**Sarah Buckley** www.sarahbuckley.com
Evidence based information about normal birth.

**Spinning Babies** www.spinningbabies.com
If your baby is breech or back to back.

**Birth Rights** www.birthrights.org
This organisation was set up to help you know your rights in childbirth. Antidote to the word 'allowed'.

**International Board Certified Lactation Consultants**
www.lcgb.org
Knowledgeable lactation consultants.

**La Leche League GB** www.laleche.org.uk
For breastfeeding support.

## KGH Resource sheets

Evidence and facts about important aspects of labour and birth.

- Induction of Labour
- Breech Birth
- Home Birth
- Older Mothers
- IVF Babies
- Water Birth
- Big Baby
- Small Baby
- Group B Strep
- Ultrasound Scans
- Twins
- Preventing the Loss of a Baby

All these can be downloaded at kghb.org/sheets and more will be added.

Please leave a review of this book at kghb.org/review. It really means a lot to me if you would take a couple of minutes to do that.

# A Word from Dr Michel Odent

This book by Katharine Graves has the power to challenge the usual interpretations of the difficulties of human births. The mechanical particularities are the bases of all interpretations, according to the most authoritative academic circles, particularly among primatologists, and also in anthropological and medical circles.

It is commonplace to refer to the size and the shape of the maternal pelvis compared with the size and the shape of the baby's head. Countless articles and textbooks have reproduced the classical drawings by Adolph Schultz. These drawings show the size of the neonatal skull in relation to the maternal pelvic inlet among spider monkeys, proboscis monkeys, macaques, gibbons, orang-utans, gorillas, common chimpanzees and *Homo sapiens*.

We have good reasons to challenge these assumptions. There are women with no morphological particularities who occasionally give birth quickly without any difficulty. There are anecdotes of women who give birth before realising that they are in labour. There are in particular countless anecdotes of teenagers who, at the end of a hidden or undiagnosed pregnancy, just go to the toilet and give birth within some minutes. Of course there is also the case of women who, after being trained to 'switch off' through hypnobirthing, can give birth easily in the most inappropriate environment. These facts suggest that the main reasons for difficult human births are not related to the shape of the body.

The best way to clarify the nature of the specifically human handicap during the period surrounding birth is to consider the case of civilised modern women who occasionally have given birth through an authentic 'foetus ejection reflex'. It is exceptionally rare in the context of socialised birth. It means that the birth is suddenly preceded by a very short series of irresistible, powerful, and highly effective uterine contractions without any room for voluntary movement.

The important point is that when the 'foetus ejection reflex' is ready to start, women are obviously losing neocortical control, i.e. control by the thinking brain, the brain of the intellect, the part of the brain that is highly developed among humans only. Women can find themselves in the most unexpected, often mammalian, quadrupedal postures. They seem to be 'on another planet'. A reduced neocortical control is obviously the prerequisite for an easy birth among humans. In other words, the main reason for the human handicap during such a physiological process is the inhibitory effect of an active powerful neocortex.

It is easy to explain why the concept of foetus ejection reflex is not understood after thousands of years of socialisation of childbirth. It is precisely when birth seems to be imminent that the birth attendant has a tendency to become even more intrusive. Instead of keeping a low profile, the well-intentioned birth attendant usually interferes, at least with reassuring rational words. These rational words can interrupt the progress towards the foetus ejection reflex. This reflex does not occur if there is a birth attendant who behaves like a coach, or an observer, or a helper, or a guide, or a 'support person'. The foetus ejection reflex can also be inhibited by the imposition of a change of environment, as would happen, in our modern world, when a woman is transferred to a delivery room. It is inhibited when the intellect of the labouring woman is stimulated by any sort of rational language, for example if the birth attendant says: 'Now you are at complete dilation. It's time to push.' In other words, any interference tends to bring the labouring woman, who was in a quasi-ecstatic state, 'back down to Earth', and tends to transform the foetus ejection reflex into a second stage of labour which involves voluntary movements.

The term 'foetus ejection reflex' was coined by Niles Newton in the 1960s, when she was studying the environmental factors that can disturb the birth process in mice. She had revealed the importance of cortical activity, even among non-human mammals. Twenty years later, with her support, I suggested that we save this concept from oblivion; I was convinced it could be a key to facilitating a radically new understanding of the specifically human difficulties during the process of parturition.

It is in such a context that we must read *The Hypnobirthing Book*.

Dr Michel Odent
Obstetrician and natural birth pioneer

# Index

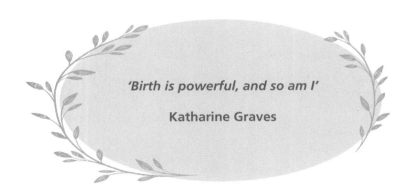

**'Birth is powerful, and so am I'**

**Katharine Graves**

# Thank You

Acknowledgements are generally boring, but mine go to a group of people who are very un-boring. The people in our office who care for me, our KGH mums, and our KGH teachers are a superb team: Ally, Heather, Joe and Lia are utterly committed to helping women and babies have the best possible birth experience. If every midwife were like Maureen Collins or Kemi Johnson there would be many more mothers who could report happy birth experiences. For years they have shared their knowledge with me with great generosity. Liz Nightingale of Birth Friend has been a source of inspiration and midwifery knowledge. Nancy Keen has patiently read through this book, made suggestions and eradicated errors. She is the most amazing KGH teacher and friend. Wendy Proctor is a mine of information for the thousands of midwives and student midwives who have trained with KGHypnobirthing.

You may not come into contact with Anna Barrington, Anthony Graves and Dan Parkinson, but you will benefit from all their work behind the scenes. What a team!

Daisy Hutchison kindly let me use her birth story, which will help all mothers who read it. Procrastination has been ruthlessly eradicated by Michael Hudson, with humour and occasional permission for time off. Thank you, Alex Drewett, for your cover design and to Louise Turpin who has Art Edited every edition of *The Hypnobirthing Book* and has supported me from the beginning of my publishing journey! Thanks to Moira Campbell, the author of the script 'Story For Childbirth'. Michel Odent and Sarah Buckley have kindly allowed me to quote from their work in the chapter headings.

I have learnt from every one of the thousands of mothers and fathers to whom I have taught hypnobirthing; particularly those who have asked difficult questions that have made me think anew and question myself. Their learning has come from their babies. My fellow KGHypnobirthing teachers are an inspiration, not only to the couples they teach, but also to me.

Thank you all.

# About the Author

Katharine Graves is the leading hypnobirthing teacher in the UK and internationally, and is the founder of KGHypnobirthing. Katharine is on the Council of the Maternity and the Newborn Forum of the Royal Society of Medicine and is a member of the International Advisory Board of the Hypnofertility Foundation of America. She is a member of the Association for Improvements in the Maternity Services (AIMS), and an associate member of the Royal College of Midwives (RCM). She trained as a doula with Michel Odent.

Katharine has personally taught thousands of people across the world to have the most wonderful and empowering experience of their lives when giving birth.

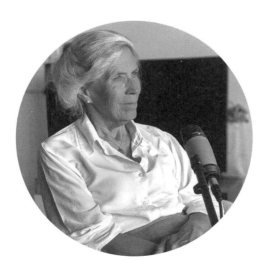